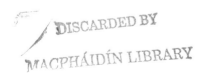

What Every Woman Should Know About Hysterectomy

Funk & Wagnalls · New York

What Every Woman Should Know About Hysterectomy

W. Gifford-Jones, M.D.

Designed by Joy Chu

Manufactured in the United States of America

Library of Congress Cataloging in Publication Data

Gifford-Jones, W., 1924 –
What every woman should know about hysterectomy.

Includes index.
1. Hysterectomy. I. Title. [DNLM: 1. Hysterectomy
—Popular works. WP468 G458w]
RG.391.G55   618.1'453   76-45747
ISBN 0-308-10275-4

1 2 3 4 5 6 7 8 9 10

Contents

"Experience is good medicine, but it is never taken until the sickness is over."
—German proverb

What Every Woman Should Know About Hysterectomy

1
The Hysterectomy Game

Everyone has a red light somewhere in the back of his or her brain that flashes on whenever a doctor suggests surgery. It's admittedly a rather dim light in some patients—otherwise there wouldn't be so many questionable operations. But even if the light goes on with the intensity of a neon sign in downtown Las Vegas, the fear of impending surgery is rarely transformed into concrete action. One reason is that it's extremely difficult to beat people at their own game. The doctor is often led astray by the plumber or the TV repair man. Nearly everyone strikes out with the lawyers. And not too many people win games with bankers. It's one thing to be worried about a problem. It's another thing to know how to solve it.

In the United States over 6,000,000 hysterectomies have been performed during the last decade. This year another 750,000 women will have their uteruses removed. And it is estimated that about 12,000 of them will die. No one can calculate the cost to families whose mother never returns home. But we do know that this year surgeons will pocket nearly half a billion dollars from this one operation. The big question has always been: How many of these hysterectomies are necessary? How many patients are wheeled into surgery to relieve genuine problems, and how many operations are done to pay the doctor's rent, purchase a new Cadillac, or finance a Caribbean vacation? Various authorities place the number of unnecessary operations at between 30 and 40 percent. It seems incredible in a country noted for its medical accomplishments that annually up to 300,000 hysterectomies are done for questionable reasons. Yet it happens year after year, and there is little indication it is going to stop.

Hysterectomy has a bad track record for needless surgery, and most American women are aware of this fact. But they are caught in a myriad of conflicting opinions. Is there any source from which they can extract unbiased information? Or does nearly everyone have some ax to grind? Can you rely on the judgment of a long-trusted friend who, after the operation, says she has never felt better in her life? Or of a relative who vehemently condemns the operation because she has not been relieved of her complaints? Who is right, and who is wrong?

The best safeguard for borderline surgery is an informed patient. During recent years, I've spent hundreds of hours on radio talk programs, answering questions on a variety of medical topics. Invariably it's hysterectomy, the menopause, and estrogen that head the list of questions. Women have a tremendous lack of knowledge, unawareness, and misconception about these issues, the result either of reading one-sided magazine or newspaper articles, listening to amateur instant experts on the subject, or having too much blind faith in their doctors.

But there is more to the hysterectomy problem than the hysterectomy itself. Some women, for instance, are fortunate in that they have merely been subjected to a needless hysterectomy. Other women, not that lucky, are repeatedly led down the primrose path by surgeons who perform what I call "knick-nack-ectomies." These operations frequently end in a hysterectomy, but, unlike that operation, the general public knows absolutely nothing about them. Yet they are an integral part of the hysterectomy picture.

Backlashes can develop in medicine as in other areas. Some women, having been exposed to only one side of the story, are forgoing the benefits of hysterectomy, although they should willingly submit to the surgery. They foolishly condemn themselves to irritating annoyances that, if corrected, would make their lives more pleasant. Others may even endanger their lives by failing to heed their surgeon's suggestions. There *are* many good doctors who think more about their patients' health than their bank accounts.

Millions of women are caught in another backlash that cannot be separated from the hysterectomy operation. It involves the estrogen controversy that has arisen through the associations of estrogens with the development of uterine cancer. It has, in my opinion, caused needless confusion, and in many instances is resulting in poor medical care. Some women who should start taking estrogen are not doing so. Others, who are on this long-term medication, are not renewing the prescription. And even some of those who have had a hysterectomy will refuse to take it, although with the uterus removed there is no conceivable way it could cause uterine cancer. This estrogen backlash is a prime example of how third-inning theories can lead intelligent people astray. Today such scare tactics have become so much a part of our society that it is essential to be as well informed as one can.

American women are faced with another dilemma that adds to their confusion. Today's society is a mobile one. It's been estimated that one in four families moves every year. The good old days of knowing your family doctor and having implicit faith in his judgment are over for many people. It's totally impossible to move into a new community and quickly establish the same rapport with a new doctor.

The good thing about hysterectomy is that it is not a complicated problem if you attack it in the right way. The decision as to whether or not a hysterectomy is to be performed is usually embarrassingly simple. In the following pages I will show that there are specific red lights that should make you quickly shy away from this operation. But there are some equally bright green ones that should make you say "Yes" to the surgery. Hysterectomy, like any operation, is desirable when it is needed for bona fide reasons. Once you know what these bona fide reasons are, you should be able to react with good judgment and common sense when the doctor says a hysterectomy is indicated.

A few words about style: Since roughly 90 percent of the gynecologists in America are men, and to eliminate the awkward "he or she" form, I have elected to refer to the doctor as "he" in most cases. But I applaud the decision by more and more of the young women who are entering medical school in such numbers today to go into obstetrics and gynecology, and I, for one, will certainly bear no resentment when the percentages change—as they will eventually.

2
Why Gynecologists Do Hysterectomies

Some people believe that pelvic cancer is the reason for most hysterectomies. This is far from the truth. Most gynecologists would starve to death if their income were dependent on treating malignant disease. Rather, most of the 800,000 hysterectomies that are performed in the United States and Canada each year are done for the problems described in this chapter. Some of them, like the fibroid tumor, are extremely common. Others are seen less frequently.

THE COMMON FIBROID

Fibroid tumors are by far the most common growths that appear in women. They occur in women of all races, but it is a well-known fact that black women have a much greater tendency to develop these tumors than white women. Doctors have no idea why this is the case or even why women get them in the first place. Just how prevalent these growths are is hard to calculate, since many are so small and insignificant that they cannot be detected. But most gynecologists believe that about 20 percent of all women have a fibroid by the time they are thirty-five years of age. Fortunately, many of these fibroids never require any treatment, and *all* of them are benign.

The majority of fibroids make their appearance in women who are in their late thirties or early forties, and they vary widely in size, shape, and location. Nearly all of these tumors are situated in the main body of the uterus, but on rare occasions they begin to grow in the cervix. Fibroids may be single or multiple, and each consists of a combination of muscle and connective fibrous tissue. Each one is surrounded by a capsule that separates it sharply from the normal tissue of the uterus.

There are several types of fibroids. What they are called depends on their location. The most common—the intramural fibroid—begins to grow deep within the wall of the uterus and is the best kind to have as long as it remains small. In this location it is far removed from the sensitive endometrial lining of the uterus, which is the source of the monthly bleeding. Submucous fibroids, on the other hand, lie next to the endometrium. This is a bad location, since growth of the fibroid causes pressure, thinning, and distortion of the endometrial lining, so that even small fibroids can cause heavy and prolonged bleeding. Growths that are situated on the outside of the uterus are referred to as subserous fibroids. By continued growth, these outside fibroids, as well as the inside, submucous ones, can not only increase in size but can also develop a long pedicle. In fact, these submucous tumors may gradually be pushed through the cervical opening of the uterus and can be seen lying in the vagina. But at the time of hysterectomy it may be impossible to classify a fibroid as one of these three types. The tumor has become so large that it has totally destroyed the uterus and there is no way of knowing where it was originally located.

The universal symptom of fibroids is abnormal bleeding—heavy, prolonged, or frequent periods. In most instances this increased tendency comes on so slowly that women find it hard to pinpoint exactly when it started. Submucous fibroids, however, may suddenly produce such heavy flooding that it results in a good deal of anxiety and can also cause severe anemia. Some fibroids may also be associated with bleeding between periods.

Menstrual pain can also be caused by fibroids, but this is not always a prominent symptom. Large tumors that undergo cystic degeneration are more likely to cause discomfort. But pedunculated fibroids (those that have developed a pedicle) that suddenly twist, cutting off their blood supply, can result in severe pain. Grapefruit-sized fibroids, simply because of their size, usually produce a feeling of pressure in the pelvic area. They may also be associated with a desire to void frequently when they press forward on the bladder or may cause constipation if they fall backward on the rectum.

A rare symptom of fibroids is a reddish-brown discharge that results when a pedunculated submucous fibroid undergoes degeneration. These tumors are usually seen lying in the vagina, and as degeneration proceeds they invariably become infected, which produces a bad-smelling discharge. However, 99 percent of irritating vaginal discharge is due to common infections rather than fibroids.

Degenerative changes tend to occur in many fibroids, particularly the larger ones. The blood vessels pierce the tumor at the periphery, so that the central part has an inadequate blood supply and begins to break down and become cystic. One type of change is called "red degeneration" and is more often seen in pregnant women. It is not known why pregnancy sometimes has a deleterious effect on fibroids. But some pregnant women who were formerly without symptoms may quite suddenly develop pain and tenderness to such an extent that an emergency operation is required to remove the growth. This operation is called a myomectomy. It is only carried out as a last resort because the woman may have a miscarriage following it, although most women can still hold onto their pregnancy in spite of surgery. When cut open, these tumors have the appearance of raw beefsteak. Long-standing fibroids can also become extremely hard through calcification. Here the hardness is due to the deposition of lime salts within the fibroid mass. This type is most frequently seen in elderly women, and some are so densely calcified that they have been called "womb stones."

Fibroid tumors may also be associated with infertility. Some women will fail to become pregnant, while others have repeated miscarriages. What usually happens is that the pregnancy becomes implanted over a submucous fibroid and has difficulty surviving because of the faulty blood supply to it. But I have also seen many patients with multiple fibroids scattered throughout the uterus who easily become pregnant and deliver a child without any complications.

The diagnosis of fibroids depends on a pelvic examination. Usually the growths can be felt as distinct masses separate from the uterus, although in other instances the fibroid may have completely replaced the uterus and may completely fill the pelvic cavity. The majority of fibroids are easy to diagnose, but at times it can be a difficult task. For example, the gynecologist may question whether a mass in an obese woman is a fibroid or an ovarian cyst. Or does the patient have a fibroid as well as an ovarian cyst? In general, the hardness of the fibroid is quite diagnostic. Yet because of degeneration some fibroids become very soft, and the doctor will feel a soft, generally enlarged, uterus. A wise doctor treads very carefully in this situation, for this type is extremely hard to differentiate from a normal pregnancy. Fortunately there is usually no urgency in reaching the diagnosis, and a subsequent examination in a few weeks' time will determine if a pregnancy is present.

The inside submucous fibroid can be diagnosed only by doing a D and C. Since I will be talking about this procedure throughout the book, let me give here a quick run-down on it. The term "D and C" stands for "dilatation and curettage." Since it takes only a few minutes to perform, many hospitals admit and discharge a patient the same day. With the patient under an anesthetic, the gynecologist dilates the cervical opening into the uterus and then scrapes out the endometrial lining. In so doing he may feel a submucous fibroid, scrape out a small polyp, or discover that the lining is too thick (a condition called hyperplasia, discussed later in this chapter). A D and C, therefore, not only diagnoses problems but also can result in a cure—if, for instance, a polyp is removed that has been causing bleeding between periods. In a small number of cases a fibroid can be removed by the D and C. For example, if the fibroid is attached to the uterine wall by a pedicle, it is possible to scrape out the fibroid. Similarly, small submucous fibroids can be removed if they protrude sufficiently from the wall so that the curette can grab hold of them. But the great majority of fibroids cannot be eliminated by this procedure. The D and C also gives the doctor an excellent chance to perform a thorough pelvic examination of an obese woman or one who is tense during an office visit. Under the anesthetic the abdominal muscles are completely relaxed and the uterus, tubes, and ovaries can be felt with ease.

In general, a D and C is a simple procedure, with little chance of problems arising from either the operation or the anesthetic. But women would be well advised to have it done, if possible, by a gynecologist, as occasionally—if the cervical opening is extremely small and tight or a fibroid is present in the small cervical canal—it can be difficult.

There should be very little discomfort following the D and C, but there may be discharge and spotting for several days. It is impossible, however, to predict what will happen to the next period. It may occur on time with the normal amount of flow, or it may be early, late, or completely missed. In addition, the bleeding is often heavier for a month or two afterwards. Patients should therefore be careful not to prematurely judge the results of this operation—at least not until they have had a couple of periods.

Although X rays are always taken when a large pelvic mass is present, as on occasion they will detect something of diagnostic importance, usually it is impossible to differentiate between a large fibroid and an ovarian cyst by this means.

I mentioned earlier that many fibroids are without symptoms and therefore require no treatment. But there is an exception to this rule. Occasionally, gynecologists will find a huge fibroid in women who have no symptoms. Tumors of this size must be removed before complications occur. Patients who have smaller growths can be observed at regular intervals to determine whether or not these growths are changing in size. If this happens, or they begin to cause troublesome symptoms, surgery will be advised. What type of operation is recommended is dependent primarily on the type of fibroid and whether or not the patient wants to become pregnant.

🐙 MYOMECTOMY

Victor Bonney, an English gynecologist, was an early proponent of the myomectomy operation. It was reported that on one occasion he removed over two hundred fibroids from a patient's uterus. A myomectomy can be an extremely useful procedure for women who have a great desire to become pregnant. In some cases it can be a very simple operation. For example, there may be only a single fibroid attached to the outside of the uterus by a small pedicle that is easily cut away from the uterine wall. Similarly, a pedunculated submucous fibroid can be removed without any trouble by a D and C. Yet when fibroids of various shapes and sizes are scattered throughout the entire uterus, it can be a very complicated procedure. In the United States and Canada there are relatively few myomectomies done, compared to the number of hysterectomies performed. For one thing, most women who develop fibroids are long past the childbearing age and there is no point in attempting a myomectomy except for the pedunculated submucous fibroids that can be cured by a D and C. Moreover, this operative procedure is not without its complications. The uterus is a very vascular organ and in shelling out these encapsulated tumors there is usually more than the average amount of blood loss. The operation also leaves a number of scars on the uterine surface, so that postoperative adhesions are likely to form. In addition, there is a recurrence rate of about 10 percent. This is due partly to the fact that the operation may not remove small seedling fibroids that cannot be detected during the myomectomy, but also because new fibroids can develop, since the operation is unable to excise whatever initially produced them. As mentioned earlier, doctors still have no idea what causes these growths.

In assessing the advisability of a myomectomy, one must also consider the operative risk. This is largely related to the number and types of fibroids that must be removed as well as to the skill of the surgeon. The majority of American surgeons are relatively inexperienced in performing complicated myomectomies because they are rarely presented with bona fide reasons for carrying out this procedure. Consequently, although the risk from this surgery is small, the mortality rate and postoperative complications are slightly higher than for a hysterectomy.

HYSTERECTOMY

The operation of choice for most fibroids is a vaginal or an abdominal hysterectomy. What approach is finally used depends on the size of the fibroid, the presence or absence of other disease, and the preference of the surgeon.

A vaginal hysterectomy is the choice of some gynecologists when the fibroid uterus is small and can easily be delivered through the vagina. Other surgeons elect to remove even large fibroids by this method. But since there is a limit to the size of tumor that can be extracted through the vagina, they must carry out a "morcellation procedure," which cuts the growth into smaller pieces. This requires a great deal of technical know-how, and most gynecologists wisely leave this operation to their more adventuresome colleagues. Sometimes gynecologists choose the vaginal approach because they want to correct vaginal prolapse at the same time. Since most fibroids occur after the child-bearing years, some women may also be bothered by a falling-down of the bladder and rectum. A vaginal hysterectomy affords the surgeon the opportunity of removing the fibroid uterus and then repairing these weakened structures.

An abdominal hysterectomy, however, is done by most gynecologists when operating on a fibroid uterus. The size of the fibroid may dictate this approach, but there is one other important factor that enters into the decision. Fibroid growths are frequently associated with pelvic infection or endometriosis, diseases that usually produce adhesions and scarring in the pelvic cavity. For example, loops of intestine may be partially adherent to the wall of the uterus, or the ovaries may be diseased and firmly stuck to the pelvic wall near the ureters, the small tubes that transport urine from the kidneys to the urinary bladder. Any attempt to do a vaginal hysterectomy would most likely result in injury to these important structures. The abdominal hysterectomy affords better visualization and is the only sensible operation under these circumstances. It also allows the removal of the ovaries, which is often desirable because many of these patients are either near or past the menopause. Moreover, if a vaginal repair is required, the surgeon is still able to do this part of the operation prior to making the abdominal incision. (See Chapter 10, which discusses the pros and cons of vaginal versus abdominal hysterectomy.)

RADIOTHERAPY

Today, because of improved surgical techniques and better anesthesia, surgery is possible for nearly all patients who require an operation for a fibroid uterus. Consequently, radiation is reserved for elderly women who because of severe heart, lung, or kidney disease are extremely poor surgical risks. It has no place in the treatment of women who can withstand surgery. Radiotherapy can be administered either by the insertion of radium into the uterus or by the use of X rays. Its purpose is to stop the troublesome bleeding by destroying the ovaries and ending the production of the female hormones. The endometrial lining of the uterus is similarly affected, and the fibroids also tend to shrink in size.

However, radiation is not suitable for all women who are poor operative risks. Large fibroids do not always decrease in size, and a further destruction of their blood supply increases the chance of degenerative change. Similarly, submucous fibroids do not react well to radium therapy because they tend to slough and become infected, which aggravates the blood loss. Irradiation must also be avoided in women who have associated pelvic inflammatory disease.

In general, gynecologists tend to shy away from radiation because of the fear that it may produce a malignancy of the pelvic organs many years later. In former years, women with annoying bleeding at the menopause were often given irradiation to control this problem. But it is the opinion of some gynecologists that these patients had an increased incidence of malignancy in later life.

Not long ago, I received a telephone call from a former patient. The wife of a government official, she had moved to Washington, D.C., a few years earlier. I had recommended a gynecologist at that time, and she had subsequently seen him every year. But a few months earlier he had died, so she had made an appointment to see a friend's gynecologist. Now she had been informed that a fibroid was present and should be removed immediately. She wanted to know why the other gynecologist hadn't made the same diagnosis. Could the fibroid have appeared so suddenly? Why the rush for surgery when she didn't have any symptoms? And could she see me for another opinion? It turned out she had a fibroid about the size of a marble in a very innocuous location in the uterus. It could easily remain the same size until she was ninety. Needless to say, I gave her the name of another Washington gynecologist.

She was a prime example of a woman about to be rushed into surgery for a totally senseless hysterectomy. Luckily, she had sensed she was being sold a bill of goods and did something about it. If there is ever any doubt in your mind about the need for a hysterectomy, *always* obtain a second opinion.

[Over the years, I've been asked the same questions about hysterectomy over and over again. Since many of these questions pinpoint very clearly various aspects of the subject that I want to cover, I thought it would make sense to use the question-and-answer format that follows where appropriate throughout the book.]

Do fibroids ever disappear following the menopause?

There is a tendency for some fibroids to get smaller after the change of life. We are not certain why this is the case. Some doctors believe it is due to decreased production of estrogen by the ovaries, while others relate it to a diminution of blood supply to the tumor. However, large fibroids rarely regress to any significant extent. I've also seen many fibroids cause troublesome bleeding in seventy-year-old women.

Should a woman with fibroids ever take estrogen for the menopause?

Some gynecologists are hesitant to advise it because they believe it may increase the size of the fibroids. This theory has never impressed me. I've seen too many women develop fibroids who have never been near estrogen. And I've observed numerous patients with fibroids whose daily intake of estrogen causes no change in the size of the growth. Consequently, I usually prescribe estrogen for the menopause even if patients have fibroids.

Do patients with fibroids ever require a cesarean section?

A large cervical fibroid can block the opening of the uterus and necessitate a cesarean, but this is an extremely rare happening.

Is it always necessary to do a D and C when abnormal bleeding occurs due to a fibroid?

It is essential to do so, just in case the bleeding is due to a malignancy rather than to the fibroid.

PELVIC INFECTION

Throughout history, pelvic infection has been a big killer. In the early days it was always the "acute infection" that women had to worry about. The two principal problems were postpartum infection and gonorrhea. It was common for women to die of septicemia following childbirth. This was particularly true if delivery was carried out by a physician. Doctors knew nothing about the spread of disease by germs and were extremely lax about washing their hands between cases. This meant that they frequently transported bacterial germs from the autopsy room to the obstetrical wards. In Vienna, when the first obstetrical hospital was opened, one in six women who entered never left. In retrospect, it's amazing it took physicians so long to grasp the principles of simple hygiene.

Gonorrhea was also widespread and caused a good deal of havoc with the female organs. Women who contracted it would usually develop an acute infection that often resulted in a huge pelvic abcess. Some of these patients would die, while others would be left with a smoldering, chronic infection. The end result was often permanent sterility and years of suffering from abnormal bleeding and pelvic pain.

The advent of penicillin and the other antibiotics entirely changed the nature of the problem. Although doctors still treat acute surgical infections and see the final results of neglected cases of gonorrhea, in most communities this is the rarity rather than the rule. Now the scene has dramatically shifted to chronic infection.

Gynecologists refer to chronic pelvic infection as PID (pelvic inflammatory disease). It primarily involves the Fallopian tubes and ovaries, but it can also be widespread throughout the pelvic cavity. In the past it was normally preceded by an acute infection characterized by severe abdominal pain, a high temperature, burning and increased frequency of urination, and copious amounts of vaginal discharge. But today most women with the problem cannot pinpoint when it started, and most women with chronic PID never had gonorrhea. It is caused by a variety of other bacteria. Since the vagina, like the mouth, is an open passageway, germs can gain access to the uterus and tubes in a number of ways. It's small wonder that infection is such a common cause of pelvic disease.

Pain and abnormal bleeding are the two prime symptoms of chronic PID. Pain in the low pelvic region and sometimes in the back accompany the periods. The pain is usually most pronounced prior to and during the menstrual flow, but many women are also left with an aching, nagging discomfort between periods. This "pelvic toothache" results in considerable annoyance and worry because many women mistakenly believe they have cancer. Other problems such as painful intercourse and infertility may or may not be present, depending on the extent of the infection. Vaginal discharge is rarely a significant symptom with chronic PID.

The diagnosis rests upon the patient's symptoms along with the findings during a pelvic examination. Generally the space occupied by the tubes and ovaries feels thickened and there is increased tenderness. The uterus may also be pulled backward toward the spine by adhesions and scar tissue. Yet the diagnosis can be difficult in obese women or in women who find it hard to relax. Adhesions are not always easy to feel, and pain and tenderness may be arduous to assess in certain women. In problem cases the gynecologist may resort to the laparoscope. This new instrument can quickly rule in or rule out the diagnosis of PID and often prevents a needless operation. (See Chapter 3.)

The treatment of chronic infection never requires an emergency hysterectomy. This gives both patient and doctor ample time to consider the possibilities. A tincture of time, with daily warm douches will often ease the symptoms and may be all that is required in mild infections. The application of heat has a beneficial effect for all infections, whether present in a sore foot or a pelvic inflammation. Antibiotics may also be prescribed, but unfortunately the results are not uniformly good. These drugs are of value primarily in acute and subacute PID before scar tissue has had a chance to form. But once this has occurred, adhesions and scarring prevent the antibiotic from penetrating the chronically infected area.

Surgery will be advised if the above measures fail to relieve the symptoms within a reasonable time. What operation is recommended depends primarily upon the patient's desire for children and on the extent of the disease. Young women who have not completed their families will be treated by conservative surgery if this approach is feasible. For example, the gynecologist may remove a badly diseased tube and ovary in the hope that the remaining tube and ovary will result in a pregnancy. He may also cut the nerves that carry painful sensations from the female organs to the brain. This operation, called a presacral and uterosacral neurectomy, may ease the discomfort during the periods. Its primary use, however, is for young women with endometriosis. (It is discussed next in this chapter.) The gynecologist may also decide to suspend an acutely tipped uterus.

This conservative surgical approach is quite justified

under these circumstances. But women with chronic PID should always be on their guard against "knick-nack-ectomies" (see Chapter 6). Too often I see patients who have had a series of operations—to remove a tube, then a piece of an ovary, and then, somewhere along the line, to suspend the uterus. This is a very questionable way to carry out pelvic surgery, and a reliable consultation is the best way to avoid it.

A hysterectomy is the preferred operation for women who no longer desire children. And since chronic PID is a generalized disease, usually affecting both tubes and ovaries, it is normally desirable to remove both these structures. It is much better to take a daily tablet of estrogen to prevent the menopause than to face another operation in a few years to remove a diseased ovary.

Does an intrauterine device (IUD) for contraception ever result in chronic PID?
The IUD can produce irritation inside the uterine cavity after prolonged use. This irritation is usually associated with a troublesome vaginal discharge and spotting between periods. Fortunately simply removing the device cures these symptoms most of the time.

Is pelvic infection always transported to the tubes and ovaries by way of the vagina?
This is the only route for gonorrheal infection, but other germs can be carried from other parts of the body to the female organs by the bloodstream.

ENDOMETRIOSIS

Thousands of hysterectomies are performed every year for pelvic endometriosis. Yet most women leave the hospital without realizing the reason for the operation because surgeons rarely take the time to sit down and fully explain the problem to their patients.

Endometriosis is a very common disease, and, although not a complicated one, it is one of the major reasons for a hysterectomy. Yet it is amazing that it took surgeons so long to mention it in the medical journals. Early doctors must have seen this problem repeatedly during operations. Yet fifty years ago it was practically unheard of in the United States. Then, in 1921, the English physician Sampson wrote a classic report on endometriosis, and almost overnight gynecologists found thousands of other cases. Today about 10 percent of a gynecologist's surgical work deals with this disease.

The term "endometriosis" is used to explain the appearance of endometrial tissue outside of its normal location within the uterine cavity. During a normal menstrual period the ovarian hormones cause the endometrial lining of the uterus to break down, resulting in the monthly bleeding. This blood escapes to the outside of the body. Endometriosis occurs when some of the endometrial lining gets transplanted outside of the uterus. It's as if a surgeon had cut out pieces of endometrium and purposely transplanted them on the ovaries and other pelvic structures. Just how this endometrium gets outside of the uterus is still a debatable point. Some gynecologists, including Dr. Sampson, believe it is due to retrograde bleeding through the tubes. For example, if a hysterectomy is performed during a menstrual period, it is occasionally possible to see blood coming out of the tubal ends. Since the menstrual flow is a combination of blood and sloughed-off endometrium, this is a neat, simple way of explaining the presence of endometriosis within the pelvic cavity. But endometriosis can also occur in bizarre locations that could never be explained by this theory. On rare occasions it can be seen in the skin of the navel, thigh, buttocks, or even in the lung. Therefore, some researchers believe the endometrium must be carried to these locations by the small lymphatic channels or the blood vessels. Or maybe the endometrium was there all the time and some inflammatory or endocrine stimulus activated its growth. Currently, most gynecologists believe that no one theory explains all cases but that the retrograde implantation route described by Dr. Sampson is the most likely explanation for most endometriosis.

How the endometrium gets to these other places is only of theoretical importance. The practical point is that since it's the same type of endometrium that lines the inside of the uterus, it also functions in the same way. Consequently, when the normally placed "inside endometrium" bleeds from stimulation of the ovarian hormones, so does the abnormally situated "outside endometrium." The trouble is that this blood from the ovaries, the outside of the uterus, and other pelvic structures has nowhere to go and is literally trapped within the pelvic cavity. Each month this trapped blood causes a "miniature peritonitis," which results in varying degrees of pelvic adhesions and scar tissue.

Endometriosis can also produce what gynecologists refer to as a "chocolate cyst." The ovaries are one of the favorite sites for the development of endometriosis. Usually, a number of tiny, blood-filled cysts will be scattered over the surface of the ovaries, but occasionally only one cyst will form, which gradually increases in size every month as more bleeding into it occurs. These cysts sometimes reach the size of a grapefruit, or even larger, and the old blood looks like chocolate syrup when the cyst is opened.

Most women with endometriosis have what gynecologists call "acquired dysmenorrhea"—they develop menstrual pain after their periods have been present for several years. For some girls this discomfort will start within a year or two of the onset of their periods, but usually they first experience pain in their twenties or early thirties. This pain normally begins before the onset of the period and gradually builds up in severity as the menstrual flow starts. It can be an extremely incapacitating pain. The type and severity of the pain depends, of course, largely on the extent of the disease. It may be a heavy, bearing-down feeling in the low pelvic area, or a sharp, penetrating pain, and in women who have extensive scarring behind the uterus, back pain may occur. On rarer occasions a "chocolate cyst" will suddenly rupture, spilling its contents into the pelvic cavity and resulting in excruciating pain. An emergency operation is then required. Certainly, endometriosis must be suspected in any woman who develops "acquired dysmenorrhea" during the reproductive years.

The scarring and adhesions produced by endometriosis can produce other types of pain. For instance, since the most frequent site for this disease is at the end of the vagina, painful intercourse is a very common complaint. In some women this problem reaches a point where sexual relations become almost unbearable. Similarly, endometriotic involvement of the rectum may cause painful bowel movements around the time of the period, and, very infrequently, bladder lesions will result in painful urination. Also, the periods usually become heavier and there may be bleeding between periods.

There also appears to be a fairly direct relationship between endometriosis and the ability of women to become pregnant. In some cases the reason is quite apparent, as both Fallopian tubes are badly scarred from the disease. But in the majority of instances this relationship is hard to explain, since the tubes are open and in no way involved with endometriosis. One gynecologist has suggested that this is because some women with endometriosis tend to have underdeveloped female organs, but this finding has never been borne out by my own patients. The late Dr. Joseph Meigs, a prominent Boston gynecologist, concluded after observing his infertility patients that women who marry late and also delay having children are more likely to develop endometriosis and to be infertile. Conversely, women who marry early and who quickly have children are less likely candidates for the disease. He theorized that the interruption of the monthly cycle for nine months in some way protects patients from this problem. But regardless of the reason, about 40 percent of women with endometriosis are sterile. Moreover, those that do become pregnant often seem to have the ability to have only one child.

The diagnosis of endometriosis can be very easy, or it can tax the diagnostic acumen of the most astute gynecologist. Certainly, the symptoms alert the doctor to the possibility of its presence, and in most cases this will be confirmed by a pelvic examination. Yet minimal endometriosis can sometimes be very elusive. The gynecologist will strongly suspect it, but the pelvic examination can be normal if the endometriosis is so insignificant that it cannot be felt, or if the endometriotic lesions are situated high up on the sides of the pelvic wall, beyond the reach of the examining fingers. In such cases the doctor may suggest a laparoscopy procedure to determine if this disease is present and, if so, to what extent. X rays are rarely used in the diagnosis of this condition, although they can be useful in select cases.

The treatment of endometriosis is dependent on the patient's age, the severity of the symptoms, the extent of the disease, and her desire for children. Today, hormone treatment is available that may preclude the need for any type of surgery. The female hormone progesterone can be given in increasing doses over several months to stop the periods, and thus the monthly internal bleeding that causes and aggravates the disease, from occurring. This treatment also appears to have a direct healing effect on the areas of endometriosis and may result in good, long-term relief. In younger women it is certainly worth a try, for large amounts of endometriosis will sometimes simply melt away and then pregnancy can occur. If there is no desire for children, the birth-control pill will often keep the disease under control.

However, surgery may be required for women who have severe symptoms, fairly marked endometriosis, and a great desire to become pregnant. But even in such cases gynecologists usually play for a little time, as some of these patients eventually have a child without operative intervention. If a conservative operation is finally decided upon, a number of things will be done during the surgery. Most gynecologists believe that one of the most important is a presacral and uterosacral neurectomy. In this operation the surgeon cuts the two nerve plexuses that transmit painful sensations to the brain, and relieves the patient of painful periods in about 75 percent of the cases. There is no effect on sexual sensations, nor does it remove orgasm, but women who have this operation and are later pregnant must be cautioned that there may be no pain in the first stage of labor. It is not unusual for these patients to arrive at the hospital unaware that they have been in labor for several hours.

Something else that is done during this conservative operation is the removal of the areas of endometriosis that are scattered throughout the pelvic cavity. This is accomplished by a combination of cauterization and excision of the endometriosis. In some locations, such as on the pelvic walls and bladder, it is easier and safer to destroy the endometriosis by cauterization. But in other areas, like the ovary, the disease is usually treated by removing part of the ovary. A pregnancy is still possible, even if only a small section of one ovary remains. Lastly, during the operation most patients will have a uterine suspension carried out, since there are often adhesions present that are pulling the uterus backward toward the spine. This operation leaves much of the female organs intact, and not only are many women relieved of their symptoms, but also about one-third of them become pregnant.

But just as there is a time to be conservative in the treatment of endometriosis, there is a time to be radical. If the symptoms are severe and the patient has completed her family, there is no point in persevering with hormonal treatment if it is not giving good results. Moreover, the conservative surgery that I have just described has no place in the surgical treatment of older women, regardless of whether the endometriosis is minimal or severe. There is no sense in performing a conservative operation with "maybe" results. Here a total hysterectomy with the removal of both tubes and ovaries is the operation of choice. It completely cures the disease and does away with any chance that another operation will be required.

Some gynecological diseases are not helped by advancing years, but the opposite is true for endometriosis. The menopause is nature's way of putting a halt to it. It is logical to assume that if the ovarian hormones can no longer stimulate normal menstrual bleeding, they are also incapable of causing abnormal bleeding. This is exactly what happens at the change of life. Consequently, if a woman has minimal endometriosis with symptoms that are not too pronounced, the menopause will cure this problem. A woman in her forties should therefore hope for an early menopause and postpone any surgery.

But there also is a limit to what the menopause can do. For instance, it cannot suspend a badly tipped uterus that is causing persistent pain during intercourse. Similarly, it is unable to dissolve a large "chocolate cyst." In severe cases of endometriosis there is nothing to be gained in waiting for menopause. Here it would be foolish to withhold the benefits to be derived from an operation.

If you are in your thirties or forties, no longer want children, and have been advised of the possibility of endometriosis, be sure to ask the gynecologist what type of operation is contemplated. Some surgeons want to preserve the uterus at any cost, and if that is your surgeon's philosophy, find out about it before the operation, not following it. And if it is his philosophy, you would be smart to get another opinion. A "knick-nack-ectomy" approach may cure your symptoms temporarily, but it may set the stage for another operation, a definitive hysterectomy, a few years later. Why take this chance if you have already completed your family?

Would vaginal tampons block the flow of blood to the outside during a period and cause endometriosis?

There is no chance this could happen. A tampon actually acts as a wick to draw blood away from the body.

Can endometriosis cause rectal or urinary bleeding?

These are rare symptoms. If endometriosis involved the inside of the bowel or bladder, these lesions would also bleed every month, causing rectal bleeding and bloody urine. But usually the endometriosis is situated on the outside of these structures, so that these symptoms do not occur.

Do doctors ever use the male hormone to treat endometriosis?

Methyltestosterone has been used for periods of two or three months, with some improvement of the symptoms. But if too much is prescribed, deepening of the voice, facial hair, and acne will result. It is therefore not used very often in the treatment of this disease.

ENDOMETRIAL HYPERPLASIA

"Hyperplasia" is the term gynecologists use to describe the endometrial lining of the uterus when it has grown too thick. Under normal conditions, the endometrium is reasonably thin, since it loses about half its thickness each month during the menstrual period. But now and then it becomes too thick and causes heavy and prolonged bleeding. In many ways hyperplasia is a disease that has the potential of being either a Dr. Jekyll or a Mr. Hyde. On the one hand, it can be a very insignificant problem that may not even require treatment. Yet at other times it is a precancerous condition where a hysterectomy is the wisest approach. Unfortunately, some doctors tend to disregard a diagnosis of hyperplasia and, going to the opposite extreme from what is done too often, fail to recommend a hysterectomy. In my opinion this can be a dangerous error.

Why is hyperplasia such an innocent disease at times and such a hazardous one on other occasions? To understand this paradox it is necessary to know a few basic facts about the normal functioning of the menstrual cycle. The ovaries produce two female hormones, estrogen and progesterone. Estrogen is the hormone that has received considerable attention recently because of its possible association with the development of cancer of the uterus (see Chapter 11). It is produced throughout the entire menstrual cycle. The other hormone, progesterone, is present during the last two weeks of the cycle, but only if ovulation occurs. If for some reason ovulation does not occur, the ovaries continue to produce only the single hormone, estrogen. This creates a major problem for the normal functioning of the menstrual cycle. Progesterone has been aptly called the "hormone of the mother" because it prepares the endometrial lining of the uterus for a possible pregnancy. But when a pregnancy fails to occur, this hormone helps to bring on the period at the right time. However, estrogen on its own is a poor regulator of bleeding. It keeps stimulating and building up the endometrial lining week after week, which not only produces hyperplasia but also delays the onset of the period.

Estrogen can completely control the periods at two particular times in a woman's life. The first is just as the periods are starting in the early teenage years. The onset of ovulation is a tricky affair, particularly for certain girls. It can be months or a year or more before the brain's pituitary hormones and those of the ovary reach the right balance to produce regular ovulation. The second time is at the menopause, when the aging ovaries fail to respond to these hormones that normally cause ovulation. These are the prime times for the appearance of endometrial hyperplasia. In the young girl it is a totally benign condition, but in the older woman it can sometimes develop into a cancer of the uterus.

Hyperplasia, unlike many diseases, is painless. Its only symptom is abnormal bleeding. In the teenage and menopausal years, the periods may have no rhyme or reason in their pattern. There may be long delays between periods, followed by heavy bleeding that can last for several weeks. Hyperplasia following the change of life can be associated with either minimal spotting or prolonged and heavy bleeding.

Gynecologists suspect endometrial hyperplasia when a pelvic examination fails to reveal fibroids, infection, endometriosis, or any other specific reason for the bleeding. But it takes a D and C to pinpoint the diagnosis. At this time, large amounts of endometrial tissue will be removed. If hyperplasia has occurred, this tissue will be thick and will have a characteristic Swiss cheese—like appearance under the microscope. In a young girl, this finding means nothing. It is of potential importance only in an older woman.

The treatment of hyperplasia depends on the patient's age, the severity of the bleeding, and the microscopic appearance of the hyperplasia. For instance, in a young teenage girl the gynecologist may suspect this condition because of the bleeding pattern, but he tries to shy away from doing a D and C unless the bleeding becomes excessively troublesome. There is little point in subjecting a girl to this procedure just for an exact diagnosis, since the passage of time normally corrects the problem. Eventually the hormonal mechanism shifts into the right gear and ovulation occurs. Even if this fails to happen, the birth-control pill or other kinds of hormones can be administered for a few months in an attempt to persuade the ovaries to ovulate.

The "Mr. Hyde" type of hyperplasia, however, can be a potentially dangerous problem. In older women hyperplasia can be a progressive process going all the way to an outright cancer of the uterus. Microscopically, the early stage of the disease resembles Swiss cheese in that dilated endometrial glands are scattered throughout the lining of the uterus. Then, as the problem progresses, the glands become more numerous and packed together. The severe type is called adenomatous hyperplasia, and here, not only are the glands crowded together, but there is also an infolding of the gland walls.

Gynecologists differ in how they treat various types of hyperplasia because there is still no general agreement as to the malignant potential of the disease. Some doctors contend it is basically a benign problem. Others, the author included, believe that the severe degrees of hyperplasia can be the forerunner of cancer. We know that hyperplasia can often revert to its normal thickness after a D and C, or even without treatment, and that the administration of either oral or intramuscular synthetic progesterone may result in a regression. But we can also vividly recall cases where a D and C showed the Swiss cheese pattern of hyperplasia one year, and then, two years later, when another D and C was done for recurrent bleeding, the more advanced adenomatous type was found. Without further treatment some of these women would eventually develop a cancer of the uterus, although the risk that this will happen is certainly greater in postmenopausal women.

Therefore the treatment of hyperplasia runs all the way from doing nothing for some teenage girls to recommending a hysterectomy for older women. I personally have seen too many cases where endometrial hyperplasia did progress to cancer of the uterus to feel confident about a report that shows adenomatous change. It seems rather strange to me that for years doctors have preached the wisdom of preventing cancer by early diagnosis and treatment. Yet here is a prime example where some fail to follow their own advice, particularly when they have no means to predict which women will or will not develop a malignancy.

This dichotomy of thinking among leading gynecologists has filtered down to the family doctor and general surgeon. Its principal effect has been to water down the importance of all types of hyperplasia, so that doctors are not finely tuned into the potential dangers of this problem. Many surgeons take the pathology report at face value. The final line will say "benign endometrial hyperplasia" or merely "endometrial hyperplasia." The patient is then reassured that the D and C showed no evidence of cancer.

Older women should therefore develop a high index of suspicion about this disease. Be certain to ask the doctor what type of hyperplasia is present. And if your D and C has been done by a family doctor or a general surgeon, you would be wise to obtain another opinion. Lastly, if you have once had a D and C for hyperplasia, never neglect recurrent bleeding.

Is the Pap smear of any help in the diagnosis of this disease?
The Pap smear is not able to detect this disease or determine if it is progressing.

THE TIPPED UTERUS

A doctor may occasionally recommend a hysterectomy for a tipped uterus, or what is frequently called a retroversion, but if so, he is most likely advising it because of associated disease, not on account of the backward position of the uterus. There has always been a tremendous amount of misunderstanding about the tipped uterus in the minds of both patients and doctors. Present-day gynecologists pay relatively little attention to this problem, as they realize the uterus can be in a variety of different positions without causing trouble. In fact, about 25 percent of healthy women have a retroverted uterus without needing any treatment. But a hundred years ago many gynecologists attributed a multitude of pelvic symptoms to the condition. Consequently, in their zeal to push the uterus up into its normal position, they invented an assortment of instruments and pessaries, or rings, some of which have lasted to the present time.

It's been said, somewhat facetiously, that some gynecologists became wealthy putting in pessaries, while others became wealthy removing them. It is certainly true that a number of different operations were devised for correcting the position of the uterus. Tens of thousands of these suspension operations were done simply because the uterus was falling back toward the spine and the patient may have complained of vague backache. Yet none of these surgeons would have suggested straightening a crooked nose because of an occasional cold. The same principle should have applied for a tipped uterus, but it's taken surgeons a long time to reach this conclusion.

It has taken so long in part because both the tipped uterus and backache were such common, everyday conditions that putting them together gave doctors a seemingly logical explanation for the pain and a quick and lucrative method of treating it. Gradually, however, when more and more discerning physicians pointed out that the great majority of women with a tipped uterus had absolutely no symptoms, its importance began to be downgraded. What did cause trouble was associated disease that firmly held the uterus in that position, although, even in these cases, it was not the retroversion that triggered the pain, but the disease itself.Women can get a tipped uterus in three ways. First, they can be born with it. Second, the uterus may assume a retroverted position after a pregnancy when the ligaments that normally hold it forward become stretched. And third, diseases such as endometriosis and infection may form adhesions that pull the uterus backward. The condition cannot, as some women believe, be caused by a fall.

The majority of women who are either born with a tipped uterus or who develop it following childbirth have no symptoms, and it is discovered only during a pelvic examination. Sometimes the doctor wonders whether or not to tell the patient. Some women immediately become apprehensive about it, considering it to be an abnormal condition. A few may also start to complain of a dull backache where previously none existed. But if the doctor fails to discuss it with the patient, there is a good chance that somewhere along the line someone else will do so, and that will worry her even more.

Although it usually takes disease to produce symptoms, now and then, repeated pregnancies will result in a large, boggy, tipped uterus that causes annoying symptoms—a nagging backache, particularly at the end of the day, a feeling of pelvic pressure or fullness for several days prior to the menstrual period, or abnormal bleeding. The gynecologist may suggest a hysterectomy if such symptoms increase and if there is significant enlargement of the uterus, but this would be the exception rather than the rule.

A hysterectomy is indicated with a tipped uterus primarily if a woman has extensive pelvic endometriosis or pelvic infection, or for those cases where a large fibroid is growing in a retroverted uterus. The constant pulling from the adhesions and scar tissue or the size of the fibroid can cause backache, painful periods, and increased bleeding.

Is it ever justified to suspend the uterus in a young woman who does not have endometriosis or infection?

Yes, particularly in one specific circumstance. Sometimes a young woman will complain of a severe jabbing pain during intercourse. A pelvic examination shows a markedly tipped uterus that is lying immediately adjacent to the end of the vagina and is being repeatedly struck during intercourse. In this situation, the only good solution is to do a uterine suspension. To perform a uterine suspension, the surgeon makes an abdominal incision, cuts any adhesions that may be present, and then sutures the stretched ligaments, which normally hold up the uterus, to the abdominal wall. Occasionally, gynecologists may also advise this operation for young women who either cannot get pregnant or who have had numerous miscarriages, but this surgery is not a cure-all for either of these problems.

Are pessaries being used much these days for the retroverted uterus?

Some gynecologists still employ them, but I haven't done so for many years. First of all, if the pessary will push the uterus forward easily, there's no need for one. There simply isn't any disease present, and the symptoms are being caused by something else. Second, if bona fide adhesions exist, there is no pessary or ring in the world that can free the uterus from these adhesions. The pessary is inserted, but the uterus doesn't move one iota. Some doctors tend to fool themselves that something has been accomplished, but the only positive result is that this procedure may have been of psychological value to the patient. In addition, pessaries almost invariably result in vaginal infections and ulcerations after a period of time.

THE FALLEN BLADDER AND THE FALLEN UTERUS

A large number of hysterectomies and vaginal repair operations are done for these conditions. Gynecologists use the term "cystocele" to describe a fallen or dropped bladder, and it implies that the bottom part of the bladder has partially fallen down into the vaginal canal. On the other hand, they use the term "prolapse" when they discuss the fallen uterus. This indicates that the uterus is gradually working its way down the vagina to the outside. The majority of patients have only a cystocele, as this is usually the first structure to develop a problem. Others will have both a cystocele and a prolapse when there is a more pronounced and generalized weakness of the supports that normally hold these organs in their proper position.

Women can develop these conditions for several reasons, but in the past childbirth was certainly the main cause. During delivery the vagina undergoes considerable stretching, and since the urinary bladder sits on the front wall of the vagina, any weakness in this wall allows the bladder to fall down. Women who have been in labor for a long time are particularly prone to develop a cystocele and prolapse. Similarly, women who have large babies or pregnancies in rapid succession are prime targets. Nearly all women have some degree of relaxation of the vaginal wall after a normal delivery, but it is usually small and of no significance. In fact a few women who luckily were born with strong tissues may bear half a dozen children without any evidence of vaginal injury. Conversely, doctors also see women endowed with weak tissues who develop these problems without ever being pregnant.

Today childbirth injuries are seen less frequently because of improved obstetrical care. Now a doctor will perform a cesarean section rather than subject a woman to an unduly prolonged labor and difficult delivery. This change of attitude has come about because the operation is not as hazardous as it was, due to improved surgical techniques, better anesthesia, more reliable blood transfusions, and the availability of different antibiotics, and because the old concept that a cesarean section is done only as a last resort has been discarded. Now the cesarean route is accepted as another adequate way of delivering a baby, and it would be considered poor judgment if a doctor attempted a difficult vaginal forceps delivery. This updated thinking has increased the cesarean rate at most hospitals and has been an important plus factor in saving many women from troublesome vaginal injuries. On the other side of the ledger, today's women are living longer, and this additional wear and tear may cause a weakening of the supporting structures, just as aging often results in varicose veins, hemorrhoids, and hernias.

A small cystocele or minimal prolapse may be present without causing any symptoms. But as these conditions progress, many women complain of a heavy, bearing-down sensation in the vagina. Others have, particularly when they stand, the feeling that something is falling out of the vaginal opening. Usually these symptoms are more pronounced at the end of the day when they are fatigued. Some women will be able to feel or see the bladder or uterus protruding slightly to the outside of the vagina, and a few of these will eventually develop what gynecologists call a third-degree prolapse. In these cases the uterus drops completely out of the vagina and must be held in place by the constant use of a sanitary pad or a pessary.

The severe degrees of cystocele and prolapse may be associated with a nagging backache. But the most common symptom is loss of urine, which doctors refer to as "stress incontinence," and there are few problems that can be more aggravating. The muscles controlling the bladder opening have lost some of their strength and are unable to adequately close this orifice, particularly when there is an increase in the abdominal pressure. Usually the urinary loss occurs with increased physical activity, such as coughing, sneezing, walking, or even merely the act of sitting down in a chair. At other times, though, it can be present without any stress.

Eventually a urinary infection may develop that will cause increased frequency of urination and burning on urination. A bulging cystocele is much like a stagnant pond that drains poorly, so that the water becomes polluted. A sagging bladder cannot hold onto all the urine, but at the same time, when the patient voids, it never empties completely, and this sets the stage for infection. This also means that women with incontinence will occasionally complain of a feeling of incomplete emptying of the bladder when they urinate.

The diagnosis of a cystocele and prolapse is easily and quickly made during a pelvic examination. As to the recommended treatment, gynecologists have to weigh a number of factors. Is the cystocele or prolapse bothering the patient? How much have the organs fallen down? How old is she? Is there any chance she may want more children? In the majority of cases where the cystocele and/or prolapse is minimal and not causing any symptoms, no treatment is required. But when troublesome symptoms, particularly urinary incontinence, is present, surgery will be advised unless the woman is contemplating another pregnancy. In such cases the surgery should be delayed until the woman has completed her family, as a subsequent delivery would be detrimental to the operation. Yet some women will have such annoying symptoms that they do not want to delay the surgery. In the event they proceed with it, a cesarean section is usually advised for the next child. I'm firmly convinced that a successful repair operation should never be subjected to the trauma of a vaginal delivery. If the repair is injured, the patient may never again obtain a good result from additional surgery. Why take this chance?

Surgery is the treatment of choice for the great majority of women, but prior to resorting to it doctors may try other measures. For example, women who have a small cystocele and minimal symptoms may be instructed in vaginal exercises. By intermittently tightening and relaxing the vagina fifty times a day for several weeks, the vaginal and bladder muscles may be built up and strengthened to a point where urinary incontinence can be controlled without an operation. It is certainly worth a try.

For elderly women, doctors may prescribe daily estrogen tablets if they are not already taking them. Estrogen not only has a beneficial effect on the vaginal lining, which in the elderly is often thin and irritated, but also helps to build up the lining of the urinary tract. Not all gynecologists agree with this approach, but I've personally seen several elderly patients circumvent an operation by taking this hormone. And even if it fails to work, it nevertheless prepares the patient for a cystocele operation by increasing the thickness of the vaginal lining.

The treatment for just a fallen bladder is an operation called either a "vaginal repair" or a "plastic or cystocele repair." This is strictly a vaginal operation and does not require an abdominal incision. The surgeon merely makes an incision along the front wall of the vagina, and after pushing up the bladder, he sutures it into its normal position. In addition he usually repairs the back wall of the vagina where the rectum is situated, as this, too, has often been stretched, particularly during childbirth. By combining this "rectocele repair" with a "cystocele repair," the vagina is left with better support.

The results of the vaginal repair operation are reasonably good, yet surgeons can never guarantee that it will relieve incontinence. About 20 percent of the patients who undergo this vaginal surgery do not achieve good long-term relief. The gynecologist may then suggest an abdominal operation. The most common one is the "Marchetti," in which the surgeon changes the angle of the bladder opening in an attempt to control the incontinence. This approach is usually quite successful and should be considered when the incontinence is so troublesome that it affects the happiness and social life of the patient.

Patients who have a fallen bladder and a prolapse of the uterus require a vaginal repair combined with either a vaginal or an abdominal hysterectomy. If the uterus is a reasonable size and there are no associated diseases, many gynecologists will use the former method, first removing the uterus and then carrying out the vaginal repair. Most doctors, however, prefer to remove the uterus through the abdomen. For this technique, the vaginal repair is done first, and then an abdominal incision is made for the hysterectomy. (See Chapter 10 for the pros and cons of these two techniques.)

Is there any way to prevent a cystocele or a prolapse of the uterus?
This can be done only in an indirect way, by a woman keeping her weight in line, having good obstetrical care, and limiting the size of her family.

Is it advisable to have a cystocele repaired when it is not associated with urinary incontinence?
It would be foolish to have an operation for a small cystocele. But some women can have a large falling-down of the bladder and still be unaffected by urinary loss. These women are usually advised to have it repaired for two reasons. First, it is often the lull before the storm, and eventually symptoms will occur. Second, repairing it now may give a better long-term result than waiting until the muscles become weaker and incontinence is a problem. It may also prevent the development of a chronic urinary infection.

Would a cystocele operation be helpful for a number of recurrent urinary infections?

I doubt that it would have a short-term miraculous result. It is, however, a step in the right direction and should, along with appropriate antibiotics, afford a better long-term result.

Are pessaries, or rings, of much value for treating a prolapse of the uterus?

I used to use them occasionally for elderly women who were poor surgical risks. But even the newer pessaries, which are made of softer material, usually cause infections and vaginal sores from the continuous pressure. Today I don't insert one pessary a year, as nearly all women can withstand an operation.

ECTOPIC PREGNANCY

An ectopic pregnancy (often called a tubal pregnancy) occurs about once in every one to two hundred pregnancies, and it happens when a fertilized egg begins to grow in one of the Fallopian tubes. Under normal circumstances the egg is fertilized in the tube by the male sperm, and in a few days it enters the uterus, where it continues to develop. But on rare occasions the egg becomes stuck in the tube and grows in this abnormal location for several weeks. Sooner or later the pregnancy becomes too large for the small tube and it ruptures either slowly or suddenly. The majority of women who require surgery for this condition will have only part or all of the tube removed by the gynecologist, but in select instances it may be a wise move to perform a hysterectomy.

It is not always possible to determine why the fertilized egg becomes trapped in the tube, but in the vast majority of cases it can be traced to previous pelvic inflammatory disease (PID), the result of earlier infections following childbirth, or of gonorrhea, or of previous surgery. It can also be the result of diseases that damage and distort the tube, such as endometriosis, fibroids, or ovarian cysts. In severe cases of PID the tube may be totally blocked, so that a pregnancy is impossible. In lesser infections a partial blockage allows the egg to enter the tube and then, somewhere along the line inside or outside of the tube, adhesions stop its descent into the uterus.

Most ectopic pregnancies begin to enlarge in the outer two-thirds of the tube and remain in this location for up to two or three months. During this time the tube develops an increased blood supply in response to the needs of the growing pregnancy. But since the tube was never intended to accommodate a pregnancy, eventually something has to happen. Frequently, as a result of the continued stretching of the tube, hemorrhage occurs, the tube ruptures, and an emergency operation is required. Some women with an ectopic pregnancy are more fortunate. The pregnancy is situated so close to the end of the tube that the muscular actions of the tube push it into the pelvic cavity. If this happens in the early weeks of the pregnancy, there may be little or no symptoms and the "tubal abortion" is gradually absorbed by the body.

The diagnosis of an unruptured ectopic pregnancy can be one of the most elusive ones in the practice of gynecology, and doctors must have a high index of suspicion to detect it. Women with this disease will usually miss a period, complain of slight bleeding a few weeks later, and develop varying degrees of low abdominal pain. A pelvic examination may reveal the presence of a small, sausage-shaped mass on one side. But not all cases follow this textbook description. For example, some women do not miss a period and the bleeding is quite normal. Others will have a period at the expected time, but later on their menstrual flow diminishes considerably. Similarly, although pain is usually a prominent symptom, it may be so minimal that the patient ignores it. It is also often impossible for the doctor to feel a small mass in an obese woman or in a patient who finds it hard to relax during a pelvic examination. Moreover, the pregnancy symptoms of nausea, vomiting, and breast tenderness that help to alert the patient and doctor to the possibility of a pregnancy are frequently absent.

Many ectopic pregnancies, therefore, are diagnosed only after the tube has ruptured, severe hemorrhage has occurred, and the woman has been rushed to the hospital in a state of shock.

In the past, because doctors had a fear of missing this vital diagnosis, women suspected of having an ectopic pregnancy were sometimes subjected to an operation. Today the laparoscope removes all the guesswork, and if there is any doubt in the gynecologist's mind, he will carry out this procedure. If an ectopic is present, an operation will be done. But if a direct inspection of the tubes fails to reveal an ectopic, the woman has been saved from an unnecessary abdominal incision.

The usual treatment for either an unruptured or a ruptured ectopic is to remove the involved tube, but, as mentioned earlier, a hysterectomy will be considered on rare occasions. Like lightning, an ectopic pregnancy rarely strikes twice in the same patient. Now and then, however, it does happen, and a second operation is required to take care of a pregnancy in the other tube. A hysterectomy may be done at that time, depending on several factors. If the woman has been desperately trying to have a child, the gynecologist will do everything possible to preserve part of the tube. This may not be feasible if the pregnancy has severely damaged the tube, and consequently, if as a result of the first ectopic the other tube has also been completely removed, he has to make a few quick decisions. Should he merely excise the remaining tube and leave in the uterus and ovaries? Or should he carry out a hysterectomy? If the patient is a young woman, he is more likely to favor preserving the ovaries and uterus. She will at least continue to have periods, and this may be of psychological benefit to her. But in an older woman he may elect to do a hysterectomy, since with both tubes out the patient is now sterile. He may also decide to take out the ovaries if the patient is close to the menopause.

A hysterectomy may also be desirable in another type of situation, regardless of the patient's age. Cases do occur where a ruptured ectopic destroys the entire tube, and in addition, the gynecologist finds that the other tube and ovaries are badly diseased. Since there is an almost certain chance that this will cause future pain and abnormal bleeding, it is then logical for him to remove them if he feels that there is no possibility of future pregnancies. And he may carry it a step further and perform a hysterectomy, since the patient can no longer become pregnant and with both ovaries out her periods will not occur. In short, it makes no sense to leave in a nonfunctioning uterus.

POLYPS

There is very little chance that a gynecologist will ever suggest a hysterectomy for a polyp, but these growths are quite common and, consequently, it's advisable to say a word or two about them.

Polyps are of two varieties. Cervical polyps arise in the cervical canal at the entrance to the uterus. Endometrial polyps, on the other hand, originate inside the cavity of the uterus. Both kinds are soft, red, friable outgrowths of the lining of the uterus, and one or more may be present.

It is an easy matter to diagnose the cervical ones. A vaginal examination will show a mass just inside the cervical canal, or it may be hanging down into the vagina. Similarly, long endometrial polyps may also protrude through the opening into the vagina and be quickly diagnosed. But this latter type normally stays out of sight inside the uterine cavity and cannot be detected without doing a D and C.

Either type of polyp may not cause any symptoms. When they do, the most common one is bleeding between periods or spotting after the menopause. This can happen for no apparent reason, but frequently it follows intercourse. A few large polyps may also cause crampy pain as they endeavor to work their way to the outside through the small opening of the uterus.

The majority of the small cervical polyps can be removed in the gynecologist's office. But if the attachment of the polyp is high up in the cervical canal and difficult to see, a D and C will be advised. Endometrial polyps always require a D and C to remove them, and most never recur. If there should be repeat bleeding, it may indicate another one is present. In these instances the doctor will advise a second D and C to check out this possibility. It would be most unusual for more than two D and C's to be required, and should the polyps occur again, a gynecologist might consider doing a hysterectomy.

A hysterectomy may also be done in certain other situations. I recall a fifty-five-year-old woman who consulted

me because of continued spotting following the menopause. Prior to arriving in my city she had had three D and
C's. Each time nothing had been found, and it was beginning to have a rather disquieting effect on her. Worried that
a malignancy might be present in a location where it was
hard to detect, I performed a hysterectomy and found, instead, a short, stubby polyp at the extreme top of the
uterus. It had been missed by the D and C's because it had
a wide base attachment to the uterus and was so short that
the instrument had not felt it. Gynecologists do not like to
see recurrent bleeding after the menopause that cannot be
explained by a D and C. If this happens, a hysterectomy is
often advised.

Cancer rarely occurs in cervical or endometrial polyps.
But since endometrial polyps are outgrowths of the lining
of the uterus, they can also develop the condition of hyperplasia, which was discussed earlier in this chapter. If a
polyp appears to be undergoing early precancerous
changes, a hysterectomy should be done.

DYSFUNCTIONAL BLEEDING

Most hysterectomies are done for specific reasons. The
final diagnosis can be substantiated by the pelvic examination, the operative findings, and the pathology report. But
some hysterectomies are not in this category. The uterus is
removed because of troublesome bleeding, and neither the
gynecologist nor the pathologist can find anything wrong
with it.

The term "dysfunctional bleeding" is therefore essen-
tially a "nondiagnosis." Abnormal bleeding of one type or
another is occurring, but the gynecologist cannot zero in

on the exact cause. He may have tried hormone treatment for several months or performed one or more D and C's, but these measures have failed to regulate the bleeding. It is an annoying situation for patients, who are always concerned if they aren't given a diagnosis, and a somewhat embarrassing one for doctors, who are somewhat loath to admit they do not know the diagnosis. Consequently, at this stage they usually tell the patient that the symptoms are due to dysfunctional bleeding from an imbalance of hormones, possibly as good an explanation as any other one. But it does not fully cover the "nondiagnosis" aspect, nor does it take care of the surgeon's dilemma with the hospital's tissue committee, who much prefer to see a definite diagnosis and generally look at these cases with a critical eye. Their skepticism may be justified, yet a hysterectomy under these circumstances can be a totally defensible operation.

Dysfunctional bleeding is most apt to occur at two particular times in a woman's life—at the menarche, when the periods are getting under way, and at the menopause, when the menstrual cycle is winding down. In part, this is because young and old ovaries don't always ovulate at the proper time. I explained in the discussion of endometrial hyperplasia how ovulatory failure means that only one female hormone, estrogen, is produced. The continued stimulation of estrogen can cause the lining of the uterus to become quite thick, and increased bleeding is the result. But the singular action of estrogen does not always produce hyperplasia. In some women the endometrial lining remains the normal thickness but still irregular, heavy, and prolonged bleeding occurs. Dysfunctional bleeding of this type usually corrects itself spontaneously in teenage girls. But middle-aged women are not always that lucky.

Gynecologists therefore like to lay most of the blame for dysfunctional bleeding in these women on the aging ovary. It's a tidy explanation, but placing all the fault on the ovaries would be the same as always blaming the thermostat for the wrong temperature. Sometimes it's due to a leaking pipe or because someone forgot to close the door. There is no doubt that ovarian thermostats do go awry and cause abnormal bleeding. But middle-aged ovaries are producing hormones that are also acting on an aging uterus. You can't expect the uterine muscles and blood vessels to be as efficient as in former years. Dysfunctional bleeding is, therefore, in part a disease of aging, and it is for this reason that gynecologists and pathologists have a hard time putting their finger on the actual cause.

The symptoms of dysfunctional bleeding are strictly those of abnormal bleeding. A typical case would be a woman nearing the menopause who gradually notices a trend toward increased bleeding. Some women will be aware only of heavy periods, while others will suffer from prolonged, frequent, or irregular periods. At times there will be no rhyme or reason to the menstrual cycle, and it's impossible to know whether the bleeding is a period or if it represents bleeding between periods. This type of bleeding can occur at any age, and it must always be reported to the doctor. Never adopt a "wait-and-see" approach because increased bleeding can be a sign either of dysfunctional bleeding or of malignant disease.

Gynecologists work their way toward a diagnosis of dysfunctional bleeding by a process of exclusion. The pelvic examination fails to find fibroids, polyps, infection, endometriosis, or an ovarian cyst as a cause for the bleeding. The D and C shows the lining of the uterus to be normal.

Having ruled out the presence of disease, the doctor can then turn his attention to the treatment.

For a large percentage of patients the D and C cures the abnormal bleeding. If this fails, the birth-control pill is another avenue of treatment that may eliminate the need for a hysterectomy. It can be taken for a few months, and if the bleeding pattern is restored to normal, it would then be reasonable to stop the pill and see what happens. If troublesome bleeding recurs, it's an easy matter to go back on the pill for a year or two without resorting to another D and C. But let's assume a woman has been on the pill for a couple of years and when she discontinues it there is a return of the abnormal bleeding. Most likely the bleeding is due to the same problem, yet after a two-year interval there is no guarantee that a malignancy might not be starting. The doctor might therefore advise a D and C before again prescribing the pill. And it goes without saying that if the bleeding continues while a woman is on the pill, something further must be done.

How many D and C's should be done before it makes sense to submit to a hysterectomy varies from patient to patient. Some women are very hesitant to have a hysterectomy and would rather undergo two or three D and C's in an effort to control the bleeding and bypass that operation. Yet on some occasions this approach can be pushed to the extreme. For instance, some women have consulted me who tell of having D and C's every year or so in an attempt to circumvent a hysterectomy. This is foolish, particularly when some of them have required regular injections of iron to maintain their blood at a reasonable level. No one can argue about the advisability for one or two D and C's, but subsequent ones become very questionable.

How much bleeding at the menopause would be considered reasonable?

Every woman has a different bleeding pattern, but I've seen some women agree to a hysterectomy who start to bleed for seven days rather than their usual five, or who bleed more heavily during their normal period, or who become upset if they have a period every twenty-three days instead of their former pattern of twenty-eight days. These are not significant changes as long as a D and C has ruled out the possibility of cancer. It would, however, be senseless to tolerate heavy bleeding that was causing fatigue and anemia.

Can abnormal bleeding eventually develop into cancer of the uterus?

Cancer of the uterus does not develop overnight. If a D and C is done and the reports are normal, this gives a woman a good breathing spell. In Chapter 13 I discuss why normal tissue does not go quickly from white to black.

OVARIAN CYSTS

There are many different kinds of ovarian cysts (cysts that originate in one or both ovaries), and they may or may not require a hysterectomy. The simplest and most common type is called a "physiological cyst" because it is associated with the menstrual cycle. During a normal cycle the small follicular sac that contains the egg ruptures about midway between periods. When this sometimes fails to happen, the sac increases in size and often delays the period. It is therefore quite common to feel a soft, egg-sized cyst in the ovary of a woman who is having her yearly checkup examination. In some cases the periods are quite normal, but at other times the patient may mistakenly think she is pregnant because of the missed period. But a few weeks later the cyst has disappeared and the menstrual cycle has returned to normal.

These physiological cysts and many of the other kinds of cysts look much like a balloon filled with water. They consist of a thin, semitransparent outer wall and a central part made up of a clear liquid or jelly-like material. They can occur at any age, vary greatly in size, and may be single or involve both ovaries. Most are about the size of an orange, but they can become huge, weighing as much as a hundred pounds or more. The great majority of ovarian cysts are benign, but as women age, an increasing number are malignant. As the name implies, these benign and malignant growths are frequently cystic, yet both types can also be hard and solid.

The symptoms of an ovarian cyst depend primarily on its size, whether it is benign or malignant, and the presence or absence of complications. Small- and even moderate-sized benign cysts can be present for years without patients being aware of them. This is because the ovaries are attached loosely to the undersurface of the tubes, so they swing freely inside the abdomen and have ample space around them. As the cyst increases in size, it pushes the loose, flexible bowel away from it. It can therefore reach the size of a grapefruit before significant pressure symptoms occur. At this point, some women will complain of a feeling of fullness, heaviness, or a dragging sensation in the low pelvic region. Others will notice increased urinary frequency or constipation if there is undue pressure on the bladder or rectum. In general, most ovarian cysts, other than the physiological ones, do not cause menstrual aberrations, although cysts that occur in women after the menopause may result in postmenopausal bleeding.

Pain is a variable symptom and depends on several factors. Some grapefruit-sized cysts become inflamed on the outside and rigidly adhere to the wall of the pelvis. These attacks of inflammation can cause pelvic discomfort. There can also be varying degrees of pain as the cyst enlarges and exerts increasing pressure on the pelvic organs. And, as would be expected, malignant cysts eventually become painful as the tumor infiltrates the surrounding structures. Both kinds of cysts are also prone to develop complications. The cyst's pedicle may suddenly twist and cut off its blood supply, or the cyst may rupture or hemorrhage may occur in it. In these cases the patient will experience severe sudden pain.

Yet some benign cysts can reach tremendous sizes without being associated with significant symptoms. If the cyst has a long pedicle and does not become stuck in the pelvis from inflammation, it will gradually rise into the general abdominal cavity. Women with this kind of cyst will eventually notice that their abdomen has swollen to such an extent that their clothes no longer fit them. In fact some cysts grow so slowly that the stomach wall gradually stretches to compensate for their presence, and that is the only symptom that is present. One patient who was referred to me had a huge benign ovarian cyst which at the time of surgery weighed thirty-three pounds. Her only complaint was that she could no longer get between the church pews. Often, though, because of their immense size, shortness of breath will result from the upward pressure on the diaphragm, or swelling of the legs from pressure on the pelvic veins.

Gynecologists first diagnose most ovarian cysts during a routine pelvic examination, and at the moment this is the only sure way to pick them up. It is therefore vital that women see their doctor for an internal examination and Pap smear once a year.

The treatment of an ovarian cyst varies all the way from waiting for a few weeks to removing the cyst with or without a hysterectomy. I mentioned earlier that a physiological cyst may be found at one office visit and has often disappeared at the time of the next examination. In general, therefore, is it wise to postpone surgery in a young girl or in a woman during her reproductive years for at least a few weeks in the hope this will happen. Unfortunately, overzealous family doctors who dabble in surgery too often remove a normal ovary without waiting. If, however, the cyst fails to go away, then it must be removed.

In the past this was easier said than done because surgeons did not have the technical know-how. Attempts to remove large cysts resulted in either fatal hemorrhage during the operation or peritonitis after it. But an operation in 1809 helped to change the outlook for women with these huge tumors. A Kentucky woman named Jane Todd Crawford had a tremendous ovarian cyst. She decided to ride sixty miles on horseback to the town of Danville, where Dr. Ephraim McDowell practiced. Dr. McDowell, who had studied medicine at Edinburgh, was a surgeon widely respected in the region. He knew there were formidable odds in attempting to remove the cyst and presented a rather grim picture to Jane Crawford. In essence, she had two choices—she could be allowed to die slowly, or he could try to perform an operation that had never been done before. Jane Crawford fortunately chose the more daring approach and became the first woman to survive this type of operation. It was an important milestone in gynecological surgery.

Today ovarian cysts of all sizes can be removed with much greater ease and safety than in those earlier years. And when a surgeon operates to remove one, he may know immediately what should be done with the uterus and opposite ovary. For example, a benign cyst in a young woman will be treated by conservative surgery. It is often possible to excise the cyst and leave in a good part of the ovary—that is, only the part of the ovary that the cyst occupies is removed. Some cysts, however, have so destroyed the ovary that in order to remove them the entire ovary has to be taken out. For a benign cyst in a woman in her fifties, there is a good chance the surgeon will do a total hysterectomy with removal of both ovaries, although, even with a patient of this age, some surgeons may elect to merely take out the cyst. But if a cancerous cyst is present, regardless of the patient's age, it is mandatory to do a hysterectomy and oöphorectomy (the removal of the other ovary) because the cancer may have spread.

Surgeons differ about what course to take when an apparently benign cyst is found in a woman in her late thirties or early forties. Some gynecologists say there is no point in removing the uterus and opposite ovary when there is nothing wrong with them. Why, in effect, subject a patient to the risk of additional surgery if it's not needed and if the uterus and ovary will most likely function for several more years?

But other gynecologists, including the author, contending that this approach can lead to either immediate or later problems, will do a hysterectomy with or without the removal of the other ovary. At this age, probably most women are past the time when they want another child.

Many will also have been on the birth-control pill for several years and prefer to stop taking it. For these women a hysterectomy makes sense as long as the patient has agreed to it prior to the operation.

Another reason that some of us believe a hysterectomy is a wise move is that although surgeons and pathologists can usually tell whether the cyst is benign or malignant at the time of the operation, unfortunately on occasion they can be wrong and the error may not be picked up for several days until the cyst has been thoroughly studied under the microscope. This is a devastating experience for a woman. First she has to be told that what was initially thought to be a benign cyst was actually a malignant one; then she must quickly submit to another operation to remove the uterus and remaining ovary even before she has recovered from the first surgery.

Then, too, one can never be sure what will happen to the uterus and ovary if they are left in place. A troublesome fibroid may develop in the uterus, requiring a hysterectomy, or either of them may become cancerous at some later time. In 1976 over 17,000 new cases of ovarian cancer were diagnosed in the United States, and during that year over 11,000 women died from this disease. Moreover, doctors who are treating women with cancer of the ovary invariably mention how some of these women had earlier surgery for benign problems. An oöphorectomy at that time would have saved their lives and seems to be a justifiable move when the incision has been done for another reason. Furthermore, the fact that early ovarian cancer is such a difficult disease to detect gives additional weight to this approach.

If you are about to enter the hospital because of an ovarian cyst, be certain to discuss this matter with your doctor. The important thing is not to assume this or that will be done. You have every right to express your opinion on matters of this kind once you are aware of both sides of the story. There are, of course, some situations where the surgeon has to use his own judgment and must move quickly in one specific direction. But there are other occasions where patients should be given some control over what is done. What course to follow in an operation for an ovarian cyst if the circumstances are normal is one of these occasions.

Would a woman be advised to have a hysterectomy and removal of the ovaries if she had relatives who had died of ovarian cancer?
A recent report in the journal *Clinical Obstetrics and Gynecology* states that consideration should be given to performing a hysterectomy with removal of both tubes and ovaries in women who have two or more close relatives with ovarian tumors.

Is the laparoscope of value in the diagnosis of ovarian cysts?
In the majority of instances a cyst can be felt on a pelvic examination. In doubtful cases, the laparoscope can be utilized, but it isn't of much help in separating benign from malignant cysts.

🐾   PELVIC PAIN

I've spent a good deal of time in this book condemning surgeons who perform needless operations. It may therefore seem like a strange statement when I say there are occasions when the only practical approach to the treatment of pelvic pain—when there is no apparent reason for it—is to do an "unnecessary hysterectomy." It is far from being an ideal situation, but every reputable gynecologist would have to admit, at least in private, that such cases do occur. This is not meant to imply that surgeons resort to this approach whenever they are confronted with this kind of pain. Rather, they have to be very selective when they decide on a hysterectomy and the symptoms cannot be pinpointed to any specific disease.

Gynecologists have always found pelvic pain an elusive and baffling symptom. Unlike bleeding, discharge, or a lump, there is no way to measure it. Yet during the reproductive years it is the top symptom, and time and time again it confronts them with an important decision. Is the pain due to organic disease or is it caused by emotional problems? This question is easy to settle when the pelvic examination reveals infection, fibroids, endometriosis, or a large ovarian cyst. But when the internal examination fails to find a specific reason, gynecologists have to start scratching their heads. Similarly, if the doctor detects minimal disease, he often wonders whether the patient's pain is out of proportion to the amount of disease present. These are very important distinctions because a hysterectomy done for psychogenic pain rarely relieves the patient's symptoms and must be added to the long list of needless hysterectomies.

It's been known for centuries that a substantial amount of pain can be traced to the emotions. Aristotle separated pain from the other five senses and referred to it as one of the passions of the soul. Similarly, the celebrated English surgeon Sir Benjamin Brody wrote in the early part of the nineteenth century that most of the joint pain in upper-class women was due to hysterical factors. It's been no secret for years that nervous tension can produce pain anywhere in the body and that a favorite site is the female pelvis.

Why some women suffer from psychogenic pelvic pain, sometimes referred to by doctors as the "pelvic toothache," has been the subject of intense speculation. In 1952, Duncan and Taylor reported a study of psychosomatic pelvic congestion in the *American Journal of Obstetrics and Gynecology*. These doctors studied the blood flow in the vaginas of ten women when they were at rest and when they were talking about very emotional topics. They found that the blood flow increased considerably when these patients became agitated, and they speculated that vascular pelvic congestion might be a factor in the causation of pelvic discomfort. There is no doubt that a tormented mind can be indirectly responsible for anything from the pain of a stomach ulcer to a tension headache to an aching pelvis. Conversely, it's also well known that when the mind is at ease or thinking about other matters, pain can be totally absent even when it is actually present. This is well illustrated by religious mystics who can walk on burning coals or lie on beds of nails. And military surgeons will testify that soldiers can suffer major wounds in battle and feel no pain until many hours after the injury.

Psychiatrists point out that many women with chronic pain were conditioned to pain in early childhood. Too often, angry parents showed attention to these patients only by hurting them, and consequently they formed relationships through pain, not through love and affection. In effect, pain has become a way of life for them, and they never outgrow their past experiences. Certainly, women with psychogenic pelvic pain are usually chronically depressed patients who suffered very unhappy childhoods. Some were abused children. Others were rejected by alcoholic, inattentive, or promiscuous parents. Quite often they are the products of broken marriages or of parents who died young. It is a natural reaction to attempt to escape from such stormy environments, and many of these women leave home for an early marriage. Yet they are frequently immature, unsure in their decisions, and commonly jump from the frying pan into the fire, so that a series of similar misadventures are in store for them. These women should not be subjected to surgery because the end results are notoriously poor. What they need to relieve their pain is a better marriage, a million-dollar lottery win, a Mediterranean cruise—or psychiatric help. A conscientious surgeon will therefore do all in his power to guide these women away from a hysterectomy.

Yet gynecologists do see women with chronic pelvic pain who do not appear to have weighty emotional problems. It may take various forms. Some patients will complain of painful periods, others of a dull, gnawing, aching sensation in the pelvic area that may be present for most of the month. Still others suffer from premenstrual pain that invariably starts about a week before the period. And now and then women will be bothered by severe menstrual headaches. But repeated pelvic examinations do not disclose the presence of any significant disease.

It is usually impossible to determine what is responsible for the pain. There is little doubt that some of these women have a low pain threshold, which may account for part of the trouble. But doctors are often left wondering whether some of these patients are actually having genuine pain and whether our current means of diagnosis is unable to pick it up. After all, the female organs are subjected to a good deal of physical abuse. The uterus, for instance, is subjected to the rigors of pregnancy for nine months and the wear and tear of difficult labors. It's reasonable to assume that the uterus is more apt than most organs to get bruised during the reproductive years. Carrying it a step further, it's also logical to theorize that some of these bruises cannot be detected under the pathologist's microscope. I mentioned in the section on dysfunctional bleeding that pathologists can't always find the reason for such bleeding, so why shouldn't the same thing apply to pelvic pain? Moreover, if it makes sense to perform a hysterectomy to stop profuse bleeding, possibly this is also a justifiable approach for chronic pain if you can rule out major emotional problems as a cause for the discomfort.

The practical fact is that all good surgeons see women with pelvic pain and they are unable to find a cause for it in a certain percentage of cases. This has always been a frustrating experience for both patient and doctor. In the past, if the pelvic examination was normal, the doctor either had to reassure the patient or carry out an operation. Today the laparoscope has added a new and important dimension to the diagnosis of pelvic disease. This procedure can be used in questionable cases, and it may help to pinpoint the cause of the pain, but on occasion it will still leave a big question mark in the gynecologist's mind. For example, it may detect a slightly boggy, congested uterus or a few pelvic adhesions, but there is no way of knowing whether or not this is the actual cause of the pain. What this means is that the most conservative gynecologist in the world may eventually end up performing a hysterectomy, hoping it will eliminate this chronic discomfort. He may even, on extremely rare occasions, be forced to carry out this operation for severe menstrual headaches that have failed to respond to all the standard forms of treatment because he realizes that gynecology is still not, and possibly never will be, an exact science.

3
Is Your Hysterectomy Necessary?

WHY HAVE AN OPERATION IF YOU DON'T NEED ONE?

One of the basic rules of surgery is never to amputate the arm if cutting off the finger will accomplish the same thing. Carrying it a step further, why should you even sever the finger if it does not make any sense? But every year thousands of hysterectomies are performed simply because women want to rid themselves of relatively minor complaints. It can be a disastrous mistake.

[The following case and all cases used in this book are true except where otherwise specified, but out of respect for the privacy of the patients, the names and some of the circumstances have been changed.]

Judy S. is a prime example of how some women push themselves headlong into surgery. At forty-five years of age Judy had suffered from painful periods for the last twenty years. It began when she developed an infection of the tubes following the birth of her third child. Her periods had continued to be regular, with the normal amount of flow. But each month, for twenty-four hours, she required a few tablets of aspirin or codeine to ease the cramps in her back and lower part of the abdomen. The pain rarely kept her in bed, and it was unusual if she could not resume all of her other activities the next day.

Fortunately, for many years Judy had been blessed with a competent family doctor. He had delivered all her children and cared for her minor illnesses. He was well aware that Judy had a low pain threshold and always felt more pain than the average person. Every year he would reassure her that the pelvic examination was well within normal limits. On one occasion he also referred her to a competent gynecologist, who similarly agreed that a hysterectomy was not needed. He, along with her family doctor, strongly advised Judy to learn to live with this minor discomfort. She did have some scarring of the tubes from the earlier infection that could cause mild cramps, but the situation would never get any worse. Besides, the menopause was not far off and that would finally put an end to it.

But at forty-five Judy was restless. Her marriage had become a rusty, worn-out affair. The children had all left home. Why couldn't she feel totally well now? What if the menopause didn't occur until she was well into her fifties? She had a few friends who had menstruated that long. Why should she continue to tolerate this monthly annoyance if it could be cured? A friend who bowled with her had undergone surgery several months earlier for the same problem. Eight weeks later she was back at their weekly outings, praising the virtues of a hysterectomy to solve such troubles.

Judy decided to circumvent her family doctor and made an appointment to see her friend's gynecologist. He quickly agreed it was foolish to put up with pain when a week in hospital could end it. Life was short enough without having to endure problems that surgery was designed to cure. Judy, with equal haste, consented to it. Finally someone was willing to take her seriously.

The first pangs of doubt didn't enter Judy's mind until she awakened from the surgery. It was then that her low pain threshold really shifted into high gear. She thought the nights would never end. And for the first time in her life she became cognizant that everything in this world, including pain, is relative. Yet soon much of the pain had gone. She was up and about and beginning to think that all the trouble had been worth it. After nine days she was home and telephoning her bowling friend. In a few more weeks she would be back with their group. But a week later Judy was again in the hospital. She had suddenly developed a temperature of 104° along with a tender, swollen mass beneath her incision. The surgeon told her it was a wound infection and another incision was required to drain it. It meant another two weeks in the hospital. That was the good news. The bad news hit Judy a couple of months later. The infection had left her with an incisional hernia that was causing daily discomfort. It was another eight months before the surgeon performed the second major operation to repair this hernial defect. And it was another four months before Judy finally rejoined the bowling group. It would have been a foolish question to ask Judy if it had all been worth it.

For Gertrude B., pushing herself into surgery turned out to be a fatal mistake. At thirty-eight years of age, with her family completed, she had been on the pill for ten years. This in itself had decreased the menstrual flow to only a few days. Yet she was fed up with having periods and she'd read about the dangers of the pill. Her family doctor had discussed contraception with her. His opinion was to stay on the pill, since annual examinations and tests had always been normal. Yet he also gave Gertrude three other alternatives—she could switch to a vaginal contraceptive cream or foam, he could insert an intrauterine device (IUD), or, if she preferred, he would arrange for a laparoscopy sterilization, a relatively new procedure whereby a small optical instrument is inserted through a half-inch cut just below the navel, enabling the surgeon to look inside the abdomen and destroy a section of each Fallopian tube with an electric current. Most patients can go home either the same day or the following morning. (There is a more complete discussion of laparoscopy later in this chapter.) But the doctor sensed he had failed to convince Gertrude of the soundness of these suggestions long before she left the office.

Gertrude had something more definite in the back of her mind. Why couldn't she kill two birds with one stone? Her sister had recently had a hysterectomy sterilization and was now free of periods. When she had mentioned this idea to her doctor, he had quickly discarded it as being unnecessary. So Gertrude consulted her sister's gynecologist, who was noted for having radical ideas even among his own colleagues. He also concluded it was hazardous to stay on the pill any longer. Moreover, why do a tubal sterilization when it was just as easy to remove the uterus?

He didn't have to convince Gertrude. The worst salesman in the world could have sold her a hysterectomy. It was exactly what she wanted to hear.

This doctor always seemed to push surgery to the limit, but everyone agreed he was an extremely competent surgeon. Postoperatively, Gertrude had an easy time. Each day her condition improved, and on the seventh day she was ready to leave the hospital. Earlier that morning the doctor had carried out an examination and found everything to be normal. Shortly after he left, she called her husband, who agreed to pick her up at noon. At eleven she was packing her bag when she suddenly experienced a piercing pain in the chest and fell to the floor gasping for breath. Surgeons who were still making hospital rounds rushed to her side. She was given immediate oxygen, drugs, and swiftly taken to the intensive care unit. But within ten minutes Gertrude was dead of a pulmonary embolus.

Fortunately the surgical complications in both these cases are rare. Relatively few patients develop a wound infection. Moreover, those that do usually escape the further complication of an incisional hernia and are only inconvenienced by having to spend additional time in the hospital. Luckily, even fewer patients have a pulmonary embolus, which can occur when a woman develops a phlebitis after a hysterectomy. This inflammation of the blood vessels results in the formation of a blood clot, which normally remains in the leg or pelvic veins. Yet on rare occasions it becomes dislodged and travels to the lungs, causing severe pain, shock, and sometimes death. The majority of gynecologists can look back on just a handful during their entire surgical careers, and many of those cases did not result in death.

It is therefore reasonable for the reader to ask me why I stress these unusual and rare cases. I have done it to emphasize that although such cases occur very infrequently, when they do occur they can be fatal. It is bad enough when such complications arise following operations that have been performed for sound reasons. But it is a shocking catastrophe when a patient fails to leave the hospital after a hysterectomy done for questionable reasons.

It has been said that the porcupine makes love very, very carefully. You should use the same approach in keeping yourself away from too willing a scalpel. Always ask yourself, "Is my annoyance really that bad? Are the pain, bleeding, or other problems worth the risk of a major operation?" In effect, why have major surgery done if there is insufficient reason for doing so? Don't ever forget that basic surgical rule if and when the time comes for you to make such a decision.

SOME WOMEN TALK THEMSELVES INTO SURGERY

Many forces are at work today pushing patients into needless surgery of one kind or another. At one end of the spectrum are knife-happy surgeons. At the other end are patients who, without realizing it, are talking themselves straight into the operating room.

Anyone who expects a quick miracle prescription for every ache and pain literally hands the surgeon the scalpel. There have always been people who have expected "instant miracles." But in recent years there have been more impatient patients in every doctor's office. It is part of a new philosophy that says, "Why shouldn't there be instant cures for all of our aches and pains?"

During the course of an afternoon, I'll often have a woman say to me, "Isn't there a quick way to get rid of this pain, Doctor? I've had this trouble for years. Wouldn't an operation relieve it once and for all?" Or I'm asked naively if I won't do a D and C to clear up a vaginal infection. And I remember one woman who wanted a hysterectomy to heal her backache. She had signed up for a golf tournament and wanted to be in top shape for it. What she really needed was a weight loss of fifty pounds and improved posture to ease her lumbosacral strain. But, like thousands of other people, she wanted what she thought was the easy way out.

This "instant-cure philosophy" is a simple pitfall for both sexes to fall into these days, and there's a good chance that if you don't know the ABC's of being a smart patient, you will end up with unnecessary medical or surgical care. Some women, for example, become victims of American "injectionitis." The monthly injection of vitamin B_{12} many doctors give for low blood, is possibly the prime example of this. Ninety-nine percent of the time the blood of these patients is normal. And few of them realize that vitamin B_{12} is indicated only for people suffering from pernicious anemia, which is about as rare as "east Ethiopian spotted fever." The next jump, from the needle to the scalpel, is often a short one unless the patient asks the question "Why?" It is not my intention to imply that all women are so gullible that they can be led astray by surgeons, but many are simply not aware of the kind of game that goes on in some doctors' offices. If they were, there wouldn't be so many needless hysterectomies carried out.

How can women avoid falling into this trap? First of all, it's important to realize that landing a man on the moon and transplanting hearts and kidneys, though phenomenal achievements, won't determine whether or not a hysterectomy is indicated to remove a problem. These scientific advances have conditioned too many people to expect miracle cures from needles, tranquilizers, and the scalpel. This lack of realism and an escape from personal responsibility permeate much of today's thinking, and it's small wonder that the hysterectomy looms as the easy way out for many.

Learn to make a realistic estimate of your symptoms. You can exaggerate some things in life, but never try to overemphasize aches and pains. You of course want to tell your doctor if something is bothering you. But if you push too hard and overly magnify the pain or bleeding, needless surgery can easily enter the game.

Joan S. was a thirty-seven-year-old mother of two children. She had always had heavy periods that lasted seven days. She had never suffered from pain, and enjoyed good health. But during her annual visits to the gynecologist she complained repeatedly of profuse bleeding that interfered with her numerous activities, and she asked if something couldn't be done about it. At each visit the doctor reassured her that the pelvic examination was normal and tried to emphasize that all women differ in their bleeding patterns. It was foolish for Joan to compare her menstruation with a friend's, who had only four days of light bleeding. The important point was that Joan's periods had never changed and she should learn to live with this monthly annoyance.

Finally, however, Joan started to push the truth a bit, and there came a time when she left the office with what she had wanted for years. Why? Because doctors also have their breaking points. They can listen to a patient's pleas for only so long before something has to give. They also start to see the handwriting on the wall. It begins to read along these lines: "I've tried to talk this patient out of a hysterectomy for years, and she still thinks something is wrong. She is also fed up with menstruation and, although she won't admit it, is also worried about a pregnancy. I'm sure if I don't say yes to it, someone else will. Since I've looked after her for years for a variety of minor problems, why should someone else come along and be paid to do the hysterectomy?" Such reasoning can start to germinate in the minds of even the most honest doctors when patients push too hard.

DO MOST WOMEN EVENTUALLY NEED A HYSTERECTOMY?

Many women have the impression that they are destined to have a hysterectomy. It has become so much a part of the American way of life that it often appears as the "in" thing at a certain age. This is an easy conclusion to reach if you don't think too much about it, and that's why it's important to take a closer look at what is behind this rash of hysterectomies. If you zero in too hard on the trees, you never see the forest.

Surgery has undergone fantastic changes in a relatively short time. Better-trained surgeons have taken much of the risk out of all types of surgery. Yet a surgeon is only as good as the equipment and personnel around him. If you asked present-day surgeons to operate on a kitchen table while the wife's husband dropped ether over her mouth, most of them would go into other fields. Today's surgeons have become too used to the luxuries of surgery to settle for anything less. Trained anesthetists are able to provide them with the total relaxation of the patient during the operation. No longer does the surgeon have to struggle to hold back the muscles and bowels that used to block his vision as he carried out his work. This often caused him more trouble than the operation itself. Blood is also available at a moment's notice. And antibiotics have reduced postoperative infections for the patient. Yet safer surgery is a two-edged sword. With its benefits being showered on both patient and doctor, common sense is more needed than it was thirty years ago.

And this is one of the problems in medicine— common sense is frequently very uncommon. Some people cite the "numbers game" in condemning everything surrounding hysterectomy operations. But it's impossible to compare yesterday's low figures with the high number of hysterectomies done today. It is a totally different game. Hysterectomies used to be performed mainly as lifesaving procedures. Now they are also carried out to make life more pleasant or to prevent critical problems from arising in the future. This is the reason women have a much greater chance of having a hysterectomy today than previously. But never accept a hysterectomy as a fait accompli merely because you happen to be a part of today's society.

Some women are also under the misconception that there is a "magic age" for having a hysterectomy. They seem to believe that during the forties or fifties something clicks into place that pushes the hysterectomy button. If they are able to get past that point, they are home free. One patient asked me, "Now that I'm forty-five, am I safe from a hysterectomy?" Another anxiously queried, "Is it true that once the menopause is over I can forget about a hysterectomy?" I also recall a sixty-year-old patient who told me how pleased she was she would never require the operation. Her reasoning? Her two older sisters were now in their seventies, and both had reached that age without having one.

Age, of course, does take its toll on the uterus as it does on every other organ of the body, and sometimes a hysterectomy is needed for a fallen uterus. But most women will have a much greater chance of going through life without a hysterectomy if they learn to live with minor livable annoyances—and this applies at forty or sixty or eighty. If the symptoms of the uterine prolapse are minor—just a bearing-down feeling in the vagina at the end of the day—why submit to a major operation? Learning to live with minor imperfections is all part of the game of aging, and if you accept it as such, you can steer away from needless surgery of any kind.

Women should therefore quickly erase from their minds the concept that they will eventually need a hysterectomy. It is only necessary if genuine problems develop.

Do hysterectomies run in certain families?
The common reasons for performing a hysterectomy are not inherited.

What is a "birthday hysterectomy"?
It's a term coined by doctors to describe patients who push themselves toward a hysterectomy when they have reached a certain age. Some of these women want to be rid of the fear of pregnancy. Others believe that in some miraculous way the operation will really make life begin at forty.

Is it true that women who have large babies are more likely to require a hysterectomy?
Large babies may result in long, difficult labors that cause injury to the vaginal tissues and ligaments supporting the uterus. This will increase the chance that a hysterectomy and repair will be required at some later time.

CAN THE BIRTH-CONTROL PILL PREVENT A HYSTERECTOMY?

Most women look on the pill as a strictly contraceptive drug. But doctors also use it to treat a variety of problems. It helps some women become pregnant. For others it means an end to painful menstrual periods. And, fortunately, it can at times prevent a needless hysterectomy.

The menopause is a stormy period for some women. It's at this time that the ovaries run out of steam and no longer consistently produce an egg every month. This failure of ovulation removes the great regulatory mechanism that normally controls the periods. During an ovulatory cycle the ovary produces the two female hormones estrogen and progesterone. Together these hormones possess an end-point kick that brings on the period. But once ovulation fails, only estrogen is manufactured, and acting alone it is too weak to regulate the bleeding. Quite often the periods have no rhyme or reason to them.

If the periods become more frequent, heavy, or prolonged, the doctor must carry out a D and C to rule out cancer as well as the many benign problems that can occur around the menopause. Quite frequently nothing is found, and following this procedure the bleeding simmers down.

But if there is a continuation of increased bleeding, something else must be done. This is when everyone has to use a good deal of old-fashioned common sense. And that, in part, means not pushing the panic button too soon for a hysterectomy.

Patients and doctors should always keep the pill in mind on these occasions. It would be a mistake to use the pill without first having a D and C done to rule out the possibility of disease being present. But it should not be forgotten that the pill can often tide women over this transitory period and circumvent a questionable operation. The pill is the great regulator of the menstrual cycle and, in addition, usually decreases the amount of bleeding. So don't shy away from this hormone if the doctor suggests it. There are women who refuse it because they have read some article that has stressed its dangers rather than its assets. Other women, looking on it as merely a temporary crutch, feel they might as well get on with the operation. Don't take a negative attitude toward the pill if your doctor recommends it. You have nothing to lose by trying it, and often a great deal to gain.

Which is safer, to take the pill or to have a hysterectomy?

Serious complications from the pill are extremely rare. Consider the fact that about 14 women in a million pill-users die while taking it, but out of a million pregnant women, around 300 will die from childbirth. Take the same number of car drivers, and 275 will be killed. And during a million hysterectomies, approximately 16,000 women die. It's hard to beat the proved safety record of the pill.

Does it matter which birth-control pill is given?

Generally speaking, the answer is no. The difference between most of the pills is the same as the difference between a Ford and a Chevrolet. But some women will need one of the stronger pills to control the bleeding.

How long should the pill be used? And should there be a rest period every now and then?

It's impossible to give a definite time limit. Some bleeding problems can be corrected in a few months. At other times the choice is between a hysterectomy or staying on the pill for several years. And there is no evidence that a rest period is either beneficial or necessary.

Are there any side effects?

Most women won't have any significant side effects. But if you notice pains in the legs or chest, severe headaches, or visual changes, you should immediately call the doctor.

Is there an increased risk of breast cancer while on the pill?

Actually the existing studies show that fewer women develop cancer of the breast while taking the pill.

Does the pill affect blood pressure?

There is some evidence that the pill can occasionally cause mild hypertension. If this happens, the pill should be discontinued.

What about the mini-pill? Is it the best and the safest?

It is not advisable to use the mini-pill to control bleeding problems. In most cases it is too mini to do the job. Also, at the moment there is no evidence that it is any safer than the low-dosage pills.

SOME HYSTERECTOMIES
🐾 ARE NEITHER BLACK NOR WHITE

In the practice of gynecology, some reasons for a hysterectomy are very obvious. The woman who has an early cancer would be foolish to debate the need for treatment. But we have already seen cases where there was no adequate reason for the surgery, and patients used poor judgment in submitting to it. Between these two extremes there is a large gray area where hysterectomies may or may not be indicated, and this accounts for more questionable surgery than anything else. It's for this reason that we should try to pinpoint the various pitfalls.

Gray-area surgery is not limited to gynecology. For example, consider the lowly hemorrhoid. Thousands of people are wheeled into surgery merely because the doctor found this condition during a routine examination. Yet even assuming that the patient does have occasional pain or bleeding, how much has to be present before it warrants surgery? The tonsillectomy operation constitutes an even larger gray area. Where does one draw the line that separates those who need the operation from those who do not? We know that there isn't much difference between American and Swedish children. Yet for every 10,000 children under the age of fifteen in Uppsala, Sweden, only 17 have had their tonsils removed. In Liverpool, England, it is only 26. But in New England alone, the number jumps to 70, and in one area of Canada the rate has reached 309. It's food for thought as to how many of these U.S. and Canadian children paid for their surgeons' Caribbean vacations.

Gynecology has more than its fair share of these problems. How large should the fibroid be before it's wise to remove it? How much pain and bleeding has to be present to warrant a hysterectomy? When the uterus is falling down the vagina from the injury of childbirth, is there a point when it should be removed? And how much urinary incontinence must be present before a fallen bladder should be repaired? Are there any hard-and-fast rules to separate the necessary from the unnecessary?

The first thing to remember is that it is only on rare occasions that a hysterectomy is an emergency operation. A woman who has been bleeding heavily for a month from a huge fibroid needs a quick hysterectomy. But normally you have ample time to weigh your decision. You should ask yourself two questions. First: "Do I actually have a genuine problem?" Second: "Is it getting worse?" These are not always easy questions to answer. Most people can be more realistic about a friend's problems than their own. Yet being realistic could save you a major operation.

How do you know whether or not you have a genuine problem? Add up the facts. Some women, for instance, quickly convey the impression to the doctor that they're bleeding too much. But if the doctor takes the time to delve into this point, he often finds that the bleeding pattern hasn't changed for years. The period is still lasting the same number of days, and the same amount of pads or tampons is still required. Instead, the doctor finds that an unhappy marriage, a boring life-style, a fear of cancer, or some other reason is behind the emphasis on bleeding. But he may not take the time to look into this detail. So be sure to do your own thinking, and be honest about it. Equally important, remember that significant problems rarely stand still. Imaginary ones usually do.

Gray-area situations that cause few, if any, symptoms

usually don't require a hysterectomy. The middle-aged woman with a number of small fibroids whose size has not changed should think twice before having a hysterectomy. Similarly, the woman who has been told she has a fallen bladder should think twice before submitting to a vaginal repair, with or without a hysterectomy, if there is no bearing-down feeling in the vagina or loss of urine. Or, if the urinary incontinence occurs only with a yearly cold, why make a federal case out of it? This could hardly be called a genuine annoyance.

It is always advisable to be a "thinking patient" when anyone suggests an operation of any kind, but particularly if it involves one of these gray-area situations. One wise professor at the Harvard Medical School gave our class a sound piece of advice. He said, "Always remember you can never make a patient feel any better if he doesn't have any symptoms." It's also sound advice for patients.

Is a large fibroid, not causing any symptoms, a gray-area problem?
If it's the size of a grapefruit, it's the lull before the storm. A hysterectomy would be in order, as a fibroid that size eventually causes heavy bleeding.

Is there anything a woman in her later years who is suffering from a dropped womb can do short of having a hysterectomy?
I've known several women patients who have used tampons successfully for holding up a dropped womb. Tampons are, in my opinion, the only good pessaries (devices worn internally), and I see no harm in trying them.

For a chronic vaginal infection, would a hysterectomy be a good idea?
It would not. A hysterectomy simply would not work. This

common problem is primarily an infection of the vagina caused by the trichomonad protozoan (*Trichomonas vaginalis*). Surgery could not remove this organism. The condition can be cured by various drugs, but if the drugs that have been prescribed have not worked, a consultation with another doctor would be in order.

If a repair operation is not done on a fallen bladder, is a urinary infection a likelihood?

A fallen bladder, or cystocele, is somewhat like a stagnant pond and is, therefore, more likely to cause an infection. But many women go through life without this happening, particularly if it's a small cystocele. Unless there's considerable loss of urine on coughing or sneezing, a woman should think twice about surgery.

IS A CONSULTATION A GOOD IDEA?

Medicine, like other things in life, requires a considerable amount of practical judgment. If you have the same recurring trouble with your car, it's often a wise move to consult another mechanic. But if the wheel falls off, the problem is quite obvious, and a second mechanic would simply be excess baggage.

The same principle applies to hysterectomy. The reason for some hysterectomies is quite apparent. Women who have developed a total uterine prolapse can make the diagnosis themselves. They can actually see the uterus outside of the vagina. Similarly, women who suffer from heavy bleeding that has not been corrected by the birth-control pill or several D and C's know something is wrong. A consultation is not needed under these circumstances.

Yet there are situations where a consultation is a 100 percent necessity. Let's assume you have moved to a new location and it's time for your annual checkup. Your new gynecologist, much to your surpirse, informs you that a hysterectomy is needed because of a fibroid uterus or some other problem. But you feel fine, have had no problems, and a year earlier the last gynecologist said everything was normal. This is the time you should run, not walk, to get another opinion. Maybe some genuine problem has arisen during the past year that requires surgery. But a consultation is the only way to relieve your mind and ensure that you are not being sold a bill of goods. Hysterectomies are not emergency operations unless they are done for cancer, so there is ample time to get a second opinion in this type of situation. It's also a wise move to seek out a consultation if you have one of those gray-area problems that I discussed earlier.

But do remember that there are consultations and consultations. Some are absolutely worthless. For instance, if the gynecologist says, "I'll get Peter down the hall to have a look at you so we have another opinion," this is not a consultation. In all probability it is strictly a working deal between friends and what in effect amounts to a "paper consultation." Ninety-nine percent of the time the other gynecologist will nod his head and agree it's the only way to treat the problem. Why? Because next time he'll send a patient the other way and will want the same kind of cooperation.

A good consultation can be obtained in a number of ways. One way is to ask your doctor for a list of three other gynecologists who are not associated with him. It's reasonably safe that he will not try to call all these doctors in an endeavor to influence their opinion. Or you can obtain additional names from your family doctor. But possibly the most reliable way is to find another doctor yourself by using "insider information." Chapter 5 will show you how to use this approach in finding a competent consultant.

Remember to tell the consultant why you are seeking another opinion. Don't try to hide the fact that you have already gone to another doctor. He is less likely to push you toward surgery because you have already demonstrated that you are a thinking patient and, besides, if he also advises surgery, with renewed confidence in your own doctor's opinion, you will most likely return to him for the surgery. A gynecologist who is less likely to do the operation is also less likely to advise one.

✂ SHOULD YOU PLAY FOR TIME?

It's a common trait to wish unpleasant things away. I've often sat listening to a teenage girl who suspected several months earlier she was pregnant but who failed to do anything about it. She hoped that the pregnancy in some way would mysteriously vanish. Playing for time can be a dangerous game unless you know when it can be done safely.

Dorothy B., a thirty-two-year-old mother of three children, was told she had an abnormal Pap smear. Her doctor advised going into the hospital for further tests to determine if these alterations were of any significance. He also told her that if there were precancerous changes present, a hysterectomy should be done. Dorothy agreed to go in, but wanted to put it off for a couple of months. For reasons she could never explain to herself, those two months stretched into three years. When she again sat in the doctor's office, she was told that now the examination showed an early cancer. Now a hysterectomy with a sure chance of cure was a thing of the past. She currently faced a course of radium treatment, followed by a radical type of hysterectomy, and no longer was there a good guarantee of cure.

Procrastinating in this way is a big error. It serves no useful purpose and could cost you your life. This patient had made the right move in getting a yearly Pap smear. But then she failed to follow her doctor's sound advice. Later on she could explain her decision in many different ways: Her mother had been ill at the time; she had panicked when the doctor had mentioned the word "hysterectomy"; she had thought the problem might go away.

Stella H. was another woman who, by playing for time, made the wrong move. During the previous two years she had noted that her periods had gradually become heavier, longer, and more frequent. She was forty-five years of age, and the doctor had wisely recommended a D and C, which she had had. Stella then listened to his explanation of a condition called adenomatous hyperplasia, which is an increased thickening of the lining of the uterus. He reassured her it was not a cancer at the moment, but as a certain percentage of such conditions did eventually change into a malignancy, he advised her to have a hysterectomy, since the best way to cure cancer is to get it before it begins. But Stella had recently read an article on the amount of needless surgery that was being done. She decided to wait and see if her periods simmered down after the D and C. To her relief this is exactly what happened, and then, six months later, her periods stopped. As far as Stella was concerned the book was closed on hysterectomy, and she prided herself on not being frightened into an unnecessary operation. But a year and a half later, she quite suddenly noticed spotting that continued on for a number of weeks. It was with fear that she submitted to another D and C, and her fears multiplied a hundred times when she was told that she now had a definite cancer of the uterus.

Never, never procrastinate with precancerous lesions. If you are worried about the doctor's advice, obtain another opinion. But don't ignore the problem. It's the same as putting something over a fire that doesn't completely extinguish the flames. Sooner or later you have to face the facts.

Are there situations when you can safely play for time? Throughout this book I describe numerous problems in which a "tincture of time" is still the best healer. But you must know how to cover your flanks so you don't get hurt. Diana G., a forty-three-year-old woman, played it the smart way. She had observed that for a few months her periods had been slightly heavier and painful. A visit to the gynecologist showed she had developed a small fibroid in the uterus. The doctor advised her of the possibilities. The fibroid was small, and it might be the cause of the bleeding. But at forty-three, increased bleeding could also mean the start of the change of life. And there was always the chance it could be related to an early cancer. A D and C was the only good way to sort out these various problems.

Diana didn't push for a hysterectomy to quickly remove the fibroid. Nor did she find a thousand and one reasons to put off the D and C. Fortunately, the gynecologist told her the tissue removed by the operation was all normal and it was safe to wait and see whether or not the bleeding would get worse. During the next few years the bleeding diminished, and many years later Diana still had her fibroid. But in the meantime, once the menopause had started, it had gradually decreased in size.

Other women who are suffering from minimal symptoms should also learn to play for time. It's important to make certain that the Pap smear and a D and C are done to rule out a malignancy. But having taken this precaution, you can then bide your time and play a "wait-and-see" game. This attitude would possibly stop more needless hysterectomies than any other approach.

HOW THE LAPAROSCOPE CAN SAVE YOU AN OPERATION

Today no book on any aspect of gynecology would be complete without talking about laparoscopy. It is possibly the greatest single advance in this specialty during the last thirty years. For some women it does away with the old-fashioned appendectomy-like incision commonly used for a sterilization. For others it is the only way to determine the presence or absence of pelvic disease. In still other cases it can put the stamp of approval or disapproval on a hysterectomy.

Laparoscopy has been used in some European countries for many years, but only fairly recently has it gained acceptance in the United States and Canada. This is because instrumentation had not developed to the point where it made the procedure practical for most gynecologists. This is no longer true, and eventually a gynecologist who is not familiar with the laparoscope will be as outmoded as the Model-T Ford.

What is a laparoscope? One could compare it to the

periscope on a submarine. It's a long, narrow optical instrument that can be inserted through a half-inch cut in the abdominal wall just below the navel. This gives the gynecologist a panoramic view of the female organs and other structures. It can then easily be determined whether or not disease is present.

In the great majority of hysterectomies it would be foolish to carry out a laparoscopy procedure. Most problems can be diagnosed without using this instrument. It is usually simple to feel a fibroid uterus or an ovarian cyst during a pelvic examination. Moreover, in less obvious conditions a good gynecologist develops a sixth sense at the ends of his examining fingers that normally points to the correct diagnosis. Yet even experienced gynecologists can sometimes be doubtful about the pelvic findings. Is there a small amount of infection present? Could the patient be bleeding internally at the time of the period? Is there really sufficient disease to explain the amount of pain? In these cases the laparoscope can be of inestimable value.

I recall one instance where the same general practitioner sent me three girls in their early twenties during the course of a single month. He told me that he had treated each one for a number of recurrent pelvic infections. Although he could feel absolutely nothing on a pelvic examination, he was convinced they had all been left with chronic infection. A doctor can rarely put a specific diagnosis on pelvic infection except that caused by gonorrhea. Moreover, many women are given antibiotics for pelvic infection who don't have infection. It isn't always a diagnosis that jumps out at the doctor. He may suspect the symptoms are due to infection, but he's seldom completely certain. I knew from a long association with this particular family doctor that he was a shrewd diagnostician. If he said these patients had had severe pelvic infection, there was an excellent chance he was right. This thinking, along with the continuing pelvic pain, prompted me to submit these young patients to a laparoscopy. All three had extensive pelvic adhesions, and two eventually required a hysterectomy.

The laparoscope, on the other hand, can prevent needless incisions, including unnecessary hysterectomies. Patients who have either chronic or acute pelvic pain can tax the diagnostic acumen of the most astute clinician. The woman who never seems to be free of pain is a frequent visitor to a gynecologist's office. A few of these patients will be helped by the reassurance of an examination. But others return repeatedly with nagging pains of one sort or another. Some of these women will push the doctor into a hysterectomy, or, if he won't be pushed, will go to another gynecologist who will. In these cases the laparoscope can be a powerful deterrent to needless surgery. It takes all the guesswork out of the diagnosis. In addition, it can be of great psychological value for the patient who is more inclined to believe what the gynecologist sees with his eyes than what he feels with his hands. In many instances the long-standing pain suddenly vanishes.

A laparoscopy can be equally useful in women who develop acute abdominal pain. Is the pain due to rupture of a small ovarian cyst at the time of ovulation? Or is it the result of something more important? For instance, an ovarian cyst may have become twisted, or there may have been hemorrhage into the cyst. Or is the pain the result of an ectopic, or tubal, pregnancy? An ectopic pregnancy occurs about once in every two hundred pregnancies and can be an extremely difficult problem to detect. Yet it is essential to differentiate among these various possibilities. In the first instance the pain would be gone in a day or two, and no treatment would be required. But in the other two cases an immediate operation would be urgently needed. Here the laparoscopy procedure will give the surgeon a 100-percent-sure diagnosis. The pelvic examination, on the other hand, has a much lower rate of accuracy. The patient is usually in severe pain, and this makes it impossible to carry out a thorough pelvic examination.

In the past, many surgeons reasoned, "Why should I take a chance and miss an ectopic pregnancy? The patient could die. On the other hand, if I operate and I'm wrong, the worst that has happened to the patient is an unnecessary incision. I can always tell the family I had to remove a cyst from the ovary, so they won't criticize me for the operation. It's the safest way out for me as well as the patient." The "let's-look-and-see" approach has possibly resulted in more needless surgery than anything else.

In genuine cases where the patient is acutely ill and the diagnosis is in doubt, no one can blame a surgeon for thinking this way. Regrettably, however, the surgeon is often wrong and the patient spends the next week recovering from a needless incision. For example, in one study 233 women with acute abdominal pain were examined. Normally, the doctors would have operated on all of these patients. But prior to doing so they decided to perform a laparoscopy to see if they could pinpoint the diagnosis any better. They found, much to their surprise, that the initial diagnosis was correct in just 57 of these patients. The laparoscopy saved the other women from a totally needless operation.

The laparoscope is therefore a tremendous adjunct to gynecological diagnosis. But, like any new instrument, it must be used with care. In Chapter 15, dealing with sterilization, we will see that the procedure has been sold to the public as simple "Band-Aid surgery," leading many patients into believing nothing can go wrong. Unfortunately this is not always the case, and I'll go into that later.

Is the laparoscope just a passing fad?
Some procedures in gynecology have fallen into this category. Gynecologists used to think they could cure every backache by operating to suspend a tipped uterus. The surgical fees merely added to their bank accounts. Similarly, they went through a period when inserting pessaries was in vogue. These were unreasonable fads that never proved to be of much value. The laparoscope, on the other hand, has already demonstrated its worth and is here to stay.

Can the operation be done using local anesthesia?
Some gynecologists prefer this approach. I personally like a general anesthetic. It is totally pain-free. Moreover, if a complication arose, there would be no delay in proceeding to correct it.

Can you remove an ectopic pregnancy through the laparoscope?
It is impossible to carry out a major operation through an opening about the size of a small fountain pen. But it is feasible to remove small pieces of the ovary to help solve infertility problems.

❧ ASK THE QUESTION "WHY?"

I doubt that there has ever been a period in American history when people have been more suspicious. For good reason, the public has learned to cast a jaundiced glance on TV repairmen, garage mechanics, and politicians. In the process many have also turned a critical eye on the medical profession. The sacrosanct halo that once surrounded the practice of medicine is now past history. Yet I never fail to be amazed how many patients still have blind faith in their doctors. They take the physician's word as gospel and never ask the question "Why?"—even when a major operation is suggested to them.

Patients who have had an appendectomy always know what organ was removed, but many women have no idea what was done at the time of a hysterectomy. Frequently they are uncertain whether one or both ovaries were excised. Moreover, if they are asked why they had the operation, it becomes apparent that the surgeon never explained it to them. You should make sure this never happens to you. Always inquire why the hysterectomy is needed and what organs will be removed with it. (In Chapter 10 I go into why it's important to know beforehand if the doctor plans to remove the ovaries.)

Doctors, like everyone else, are pressed for time these days. Consequently, don't expect a long-drawn-out explanation. What you want is a concise, logical reason for your surgery. This is sometimes easier said than done. Many patients have doctors who are "nontalkers." They may be excellent physicians, but have never learned the ABC's of communication. You can't change their personalities, but you can drag the pertinent information out of them by short, pointed questions. Why is the surgery needed? What will happen if the operation is postponed? Would it be dangerous to delay? Will the condition get worse? Could it change into a cancer? Does the doctor plan to take out the ovaries? Does he normally remove the appendix during a hysterectomy?

This approach will quickly determine why you need a hysterectomy. Surely, if it's sound practice to ask a garage mechanic why you need the repairs on your car, it behooves you to be more inquisitive about your own body.

After surgery, is it advisable to ask for a copy of the operative report?

You don't have to go that far, since it is usually difficult for a layman to understand such reports. Just make sure that, following any operation, you are told what was removed and what was done.

Is it best to have the appendix removed during a hysterectomy?

A good number of surgeons prefer to take it out. Others routinely leave it in unless the appendix appears to be diseased. "Let's-leave-it-in" surgeons reason that removing it adds a small additional risk to the operation, and why should they assume even this exceedingly small danger when so many patients are suing doctors these days? If you have a preference, you should discuss it with the surgeon prior to the operation.

Would removing the appendix increase the pain following a hysterectomy?

The additional surgery would have no noticeable effect on the pain.

4
Why Do Surgeons Perform Needless Hysterectomies?

Life, in so many ways, is a game of chance. What happens to us often hinges on luck rather than good planning. The hysterectomy operation is no exception. For instance, it may come as a surprise that where you happen to live determines, in part, your chances of having this operation.

✖ GEOGRAPHY AND MONEY

Dr. John Vennberg of Harvard University and Dr. Alan Gettlesohn of the Johns Hopkins School of Hygiene and Public Health found that the surgical rates for hysterectomy varied considerably even within the same state. For example, some parts of Vermont had rates three times higher than others. The National Center for Health Statisticts reports that 10 percent more hysterectomies are performed in the South than in the Northeast, and 50 percent more than in the West. On a world scale there are also some interesting statistics. U.S. women are four times more likely to undergo this operation than Swedish women, and two and a half times more likely than English women.

Why should there be such variations in the United States? It is hard to conclude that either the mountains of Vermont or the heat of Alabama has any effect on the uterus. Most authorities point to two factors: the number of surgeons in a particular area and the kind of medical insurance plan the patient has. In some parts of the United States there are too many gynecologists at a time when the birth rate is declining. Young surgeons run into stiff competition, and older ones see their overhead rising sharply in these inflationary times.

A general rule of thumb has traditionally held that one gynecologist can be supported by about fifteen thousand patients. But this is because nearly all of them also do obstetrics. During the last decade the birth-control pill has cut deeply into this part of their practice. This old rule has therefore become obsolete. There is also another factor that continues to be more important than the pill. Gynecologists, except for those in teaching hospitals, have never had the field of gynecology to themselves. General surgeons were the first on the scene and continue to do their fair share of pelvic surgery. In addition, in some hospitals a certain number of family doctors tend to dabble in this kind of surgery. Consequently, even under the best of conditions some gynecologists seem to be always looking for more surgery. In such a highly competitive area, too often the uterus may be removed to pay the rent.

The role played by insurance is even easier to nail

down. An insured woman has twice the chance of having a hysterectomy that an uninsured one has. But the real shock wave hits when you realize that some insurance plans protect you, and other kinds are inclined to push you toward surgery. It has been shown that women who have the fee-for-service plans such as Blue Cross—Blue Shield have a greater chance of having a hysterectomy than women who are members of prepaid plans run by groups such as the Kaiser Foundation.

Why should a plan like Kaiser's control the number of needless hysterectomies? A number of factors come into play. The surgeons are on a salary and have nothing to gain by adding to their work load. Conversely, the foundation has something to lose if too much surgery is performed and operating costs increase. Moreover, to make certain a knife-happy surgeon isn't in their midst, peer-review studies are carried out on all hysterectomies. Some peer-review studies in other hospitals don't have much teeth. A member of the committee may take the offending surgeon aside and say, "Sam, we think you're doing too many questionable hysterectomies. How about easing up a bit?" Sam may do so temporarily, but usually he's back on the same old merry-go-round before too long. But in a controlled situation like Kaiser's, the hand of restraint can descend quickly and heavily on an overzealous surgeon.

The low rate of hysterectomy in England and Sweden can be explained in much the same way. Under nationalized medicine there is no additional financial gain from doing another hysterectomy. I once attended a meeting of the Royal College of Obstetricians and Gynecologists in London, England, and spent an afternoon observing surgery at Guy's Hospital. The attending gynecologist complained bitterly to me that for his hour of work he would receive the princely sum of two pounds, the equivalent of four U.S. dollars.

For the fee-for-service surgeon, money and inflation can have a strong influence over the decision of whether or not to operate. Seeing a potential six-hundred-dollar hysterectomy patient sitting on the other side of the desk, such a gynecologist cannot totally exclude money from his thinking. This is why some highly respected surgeons have called for the complete abolition of the fee-for-service concept. Dr. George Crile, emeritus consultant in surgery at the Cleveland Clinic, is an outspoken advocate of this approach. He, like many others, is convinced that the fee-for-service surgeon must constantly grapple with this conflict of interest every time he weighs the pros and cons of surgery. If the surgeon operates, he gets a fat fee. If he decides against it, he receives nothing. The implications are obvious if the surgeon has a borderline conscience.

Since most Americans and Canadians go to fee-for-service gynecologists, there is a strong suspicion that it is money that accounts primarily for the bulk of needless hysterectomies. U.S. surgeons argue in their defense that there is too little surgery done in countries like England and Sweden. They say that British gynecologists bypass needed surgery because there is no financial incentive. And that English women suffer because of it. This may be true in part. But if, for example, women in England were being deprived of essential surgery in gallbladder disease, then the death rate from this problem would be higher than in other countries. But one study showed that Canadians have a higher mortality rate from gallbladder disease than the English. And some of this excess mortality may be the result of surgery.

Much of the strength of the United States has derived from the capitalistic free-enterprise system. But when high surgical fees are guaranteed by a variety of insurance schemes, much of the controlling sting is removed from this competitive environment. It's for this reason that women should keep the "money game" foremost in their minds when any surgeon talks quickly about the advantages of the hysterectomy operation.

WE ALL LIKE TO BE "TOP BANANA"

Some hysterectomies are done strictly to satisfy a gynecologist's ego. Everyone likes to be tops in his field, whether it's baseball, hockey, or surgery. Big-name athletes are applauded because their talent is obvious to millions of TV fans, but they can't hide their age and decreasing skills from the same exposure. Astute managers and the increasing boos of the onlookers are good controls as to how long they can play the game.

Gynecologists, on the other hand, are on display in a much more subtle way. For instance, no one is aware of the daily number of electrocardiograms read by a specialist in internal medicine. Similarly, the hospital staff would have no idea, nor would they care, how many allergy tests were being done by a dermatologist. Yet the hospital personnel do focus in on surgery. They can easily estimate the popularity of a surgeon, simply by checking the operating lists that are posted throughout the hospital. Day after day these lists spell out the story of who is doing what in the OR. Surgeons, by and large, are a rather outgoing group compared with many of the other specialists. It's therefore natural that each one wants to be known as one of the "big guns." Young surgeons want to edge their way onto these OR lists. Older ones don't want to be pushed off them. One can't ignore the surgeon's psyche when trying to explain the vast number of questionable hysterectomies.

U.S. surgeons have a worldwide reputation as "aggressive cutters." Some critics explain it strictly on the basis of money, but that is just part of the story. The tremendous egomania of some surgeons requires that they have long operating lists. This "high-volume complex" can occur at any age. But when a surgeon starts to slide down the list because of advancing age, he may try to hang in there by doing more "gray-area surgery."

I mention this aspect of unnecessary surgery because some women get trapped by it. They go to a particular gynecologist because they hear he is the busiest one in town. This may indicate that he is the best one in the community, but it may also indicate that he is a questionable, high-volume operator and one to shy away from. The person on the street has no way of knowing who is busy performing necessary surgery and who is merely bolstering his own ego. That is why it is so important to choose a competent gynecologist. (See Chapter 5.)

REFERRING DOCTORS
CAN CAUSE TROUBLE

There is no substitute for a good family doctor in today's complicated medical maze. He can steer you away from many types of questionable treatments. His ability to look at the forest as well as the trees is an invaluable asset. But some general practitioners also have a "let's-cut-it-out" approach in dealing with the uterus. It's an attitude that may have more momentum in getting you on the operating table than even the efforts of an eager gynecologist.

In every hospital, gynecologists and general surgeons have their own network of referring doctors. Why one GP routinely sends his patients to a particular surgeon is often very difficult to assess. He may consider him the best surgeon for that operation. Or it may be because he's a speedy gynecologist and doesn't waste all morning doing one case. Most GP's don't like being tied up in the OR too long, as it interferes with their other work. Or it may just be because he's a good golf partner, belongs to the same church or club, or has an office in the same building. And in some instances it merely becomes a matter of habit. But the reason for the referral isn't the important point. What is of consequence is that specialists like to keep referring doctors happy.

Let's assume that in the course of one week Dr. A. refers a couple of cases to Dr. B. for hysterectomies. But it turns out that Dr. B. doesn't feel that the indications are sufficient for the operation. In some instances this isn't a problem. The specialist knows from past experience that turning these cases down won't severely jar the referring doctor's psyche. But it's not always that easy. Some family physicians have very fragile feelings. They may already have told the patient in no uncertain terms that an operation is the best treatment. It annoys and embarrasses them if the patient is later told otherwise. Specialists develop a sixth sense for this type of situation and in borderline cases may go along with the GP's advice. Failure to do so could mean that another specialist will be called in for the next patient.

The moral of the story is: Don't push any doctor toward a hysterectomy, even your family doctor. He may, without your knowing it, be your last line of defense.

5
How to Choose a Competent Gynecologist

Recently I've noticed a new trend in the kinds of questions I'm asked on radio talk shows. Women—who have become more consumer-conscious in medicine as in other areas—are now asking: "How can I pick a good gynecologist?" and "Is there any way I can evaluate the surgeon who is to perform my hysterectomy?"

As I will show you, it's easier to determine who's who in surgery than it is to evaluate who is a good TV repairman or a good auto mechanic, even though so many people do it the wrong way and end up with inferior and potentially dangerous surgical care. Never forget that it is the surgeon who is the kingpin in settling whether or not you receive superior treatment. It is not the hospital, nor is it the fancy laboratory tests.

DON'T RELY
ON THE YELLOW PAGES

Occasionally patients tell me they picked me out of the Yellow Pages of the telephone book. I'm never too sure how to react to this remark. Maybe my name reminded them of a great-uncle, or possibly they just liked the sound of it. But usually I find I was only a chance selection. This Russian roulette way of choosing a gynecologist, or any other doctor, is fraught with danger.

The telephone company stresses that the Yellow Pages are a good place to find most things. It's therefore a natural reaction for some people to turn to this section, for surely if a gynecologist's name is listed there, he or she must be a reliable doctor.

You may be on reasonably safe ground if you use these pages to find a TV set or an Afghan rug. But never, never resort to this method for your medical care. The Consumer Protection Council recently discovered that 7 to 13 percent of the doctors listed in the Yellow Pages of the New York telephone directory were not licensed to practice medicine in New York State. They were chiropractors, or unlicensed graduates of foreign medical schools, or had no apparent qualifications at all. All anyone had to do to be listed was send in their money. The telephone company had a "good-faith" policy and had been playing the game that way for many years.

Fortunately the telephone company put an end to this policy and now checks with the local medical society before publishing a doctor's name. Yet this merely proves a doctor is a doctor. One can hardly expect the telephone company to rate doctors. Even medical schools have a fairly hard job doing this. Happily, few doctors in the United States are outright incompetents. Most likely you wouldn't hit one by running your fingers down those Yellow Pages, but there is a reasonable chance you might hit one of the "gray-area" gynecologists. You might end up with one who X rays you from head to toe at the drop of a hat. Or one who routinely orders a list of lab tests as long as your arm. Sometimes it's done to impress you. At other times it's done because of the doctor's diagnostic insecurity. You don't want that kind of gynecologist.

🍳 GOSSIP CAN LEAD YOU ASTRAY

Just as the Yellow Pages can lead you down the wrong path, gossip can take you a step farther in the wrong direction. Yet many women rely on it, particularly if they have moved to a new location and are looking for a doctor in the area. Without checking further, they will listen to a next-door neighbor, or someone at church or at the office. This is a way to get your fingers burned, and if you don't, it's only because Lady Luck is on your side.

Jeanne B. was one of those who ran out of luck. She had lived all her life in New York before moving with her family to a small Midwestern town. She had seen her gynecologist just prior to leaving, and at that time she had learned that a small fibroid was present, which explained her increased bleeding for several months. Now everything seemed to be going wrong. Her husband was unhappy in his new job. The children were homesick for their old friends and school. And Jeanne found it difficult adjusting to the life of a small town. She was also worried about the bleeding. Since the move she had been bleeding nearly every day. At one point she considered flying back to New York to see her gynecologist. But making a trip East didn't seem practical. She mentioned her problem to her next-door neighbor, who recommended her own family doctor. He had been her doctor and father-confessor for years, and he had performed a hysterectomy on her several years earlier.

A week later Jeanne was in his office. He agreed she had a fibroid and told her a hysterectomy was the only way to stop the bleeding. Jeanne had too many other problems on her mind to give much thought to it. A few days later she was admitted to the local hospital, grateful the doctor could arrange it so quickly. Her main desire was to get rid of a constant annoyance and then get back to other pressing matters.

Doctor X. was a sound general practitioner and over the years had obtained operating privileges for some surgery, such as hysterectomy. He also had a good track record. If he sensed something difficult, he would refer the case to a qualified surgeon. But Jeanne's uterus was small, and the fibroid seemed to be no larger than a plum. So it should have been a simple job to take it out.

The first suggestion of trouble loomed when he opened the abdomen. The uterus was normal in size, but the tumor was larger than he had previously thought. Its location spelled trouble. It was buried deep in the pelvic cavity, down near the opening of the uterus. This brought it close to some extremely vital structures, one being the ureter that carries the urine from the kidney to the bladder. At this point he should quickly have put in a call to one of the gynecologists. But that would have meant losing a considerable amount of face with everyone.

Initially the operation went easily. Then, as he penetrated more deeply into the area around the fibroid, he encountered extensive bleeding. Suddenly the pelvic cavity was full of blood and he could not be certain of the source of the hemorrhage. He repeatedly placed and replaced clamps in the general vicinity of the uterine arteries, but this failed to control all of the bleeding. Finally, he placed a larger hemostat deeper into the cavity of the pelvis. The hemorrhage stopped, and he quickly tied off the large bundles of tissue containing the uterine vessels and removed the fibroid uterus.

Yet Jeanne's trouble had just begun. In his frantic efforts to clamp the uterine vessels, his blind probing had also tied off the ureter on one side. It was a catastrophic error. Several days later Jeanne suddenly developed a temperature of 104°, severe pain in her right back, along with nausea and vomiting. She was placed on large doses of antibiotics, but twenty-four hours later her condition had worsened. Finally a consultant was called in, and X rays showed a complete blockage of the right ureter. An emergency operation to repair the urinary tube was required. This is always a difficult task because the tissues are swollen from the previous operation and bleed easily. Moreover, because of the injury, scar tissue can form around the ureter, causing later problems. Jeanne was finally discharged, but she had no guarantee as to what her future might hold.

Napoleon once said, "In order to have a good army, a nation must always be at war." The same basic principle applies to surgery—you must operate continually to retain your technical skill. A well-trained gynecologist can, of course, injure a ureter during the course of his lifetime. But his batting average is considerably better than that of the doctor who now and then dabbles in surgery. Thousands of women spend more time in buying a dress than in deciding who is going to perform a major operation on them. Don't rely wholly on advice you get from someone you don't know well—not when it concerns your health.

DON'T ALLOW THE FAMILY DOCTOR 🦋 TO PERFORM THE HYSTERECTOMY

Although the general practitioner-surgeon is gradually dying out in the United States and Canada, the number still operating in many communities makes the inclusion of the topic in this book important. There is no doubt that in the past these doctors performed a much-needed role. And in certain areas today, patients would be in trouble without them. I also hasten to add that some of these self-trained surgeons become excellent technicians. But looking at the total picture, surgeons who have gone through the long years of training should get the first nod from patients. Surgery is just like any other game. The more you can cut down the odds, the greater the chance of winning.

How do you tell your family doctor, a man you've known and respected for years, perhaps, that you don't want him to do the operation? It's obviously difficult and often embarrassing for most people. The best way to start is to ask for a consultation. It's reasonable to say to your doctor that you are concerned about having a hysterectomy and would like another opinion. Any doctor who balks at such a request becomes highly suspect. So let's assume he goes along with it, and the consultant agrees that the operation is required.

At this point, you have to make the final move. You have to make clear to your family doctor that in this day and age you would prefer the surgery to be done by a specialist. You can also get yourself off the hook by saying another member of the family would feel happier if this were done. Don't get into a game of comparisons between him and the other doctor. This would be unkind to a man who has done a good job of caring for you and your family for many years.

Just in case you still have pangs of doubt, remember one other thing. Doctors always run to top-drawer surgeons whenever they themselves need an operation. So what's good for your doctor is equally good for you. And it may seem obvious why doctors pick out a certain surgeon, but there's a good chance you're thinking of the wrong reason. It's not because the surgeon is smart. Doctors ask only one question about a surgeon: Does he have skilled hands?

The majority of gynecological and other diseases that call for surgery are not that difficult to diagnose. For example, let's assume that a woman has noticed some rectal bleeding. In the great majority of cases it's due to hemorrhoids, but if it's caused by cancer, the diagnosis is made in two ways. First, a lighted instrument called the sigmoidoscope is inserted into the rectum to visualize the tumor. Second, X rays are taken to detect tumors out of reach of this instrument. This doesn't take much skill or brilliance. Similarly, if the patient has a falling-down of the uterus, the trouble is quite obvious. Even the patient can make the diagnosis. Therefore, it is the surgeon's hands that are all-important. In most cases, they can all come up with the same diagnosis, but there are great differences in their technical abilities. For your operation, you want the doctor whose primary training is surgery.

HOW TO OBTAIN
"INSIDER INFORMATION"

There are many sources that can lead you to a competent gynecologist. But for most people living in a large city a nurse is the ideal choice. Day after day nurses have constant contact with both family doctors and specialists. Yet some people have the impression that it's unethical for nurses to say who is good and who is bad. It's the wrong notion. Most nurses are more than willing to steer women in the right direction. Good nurses have a high regard for proper medical care and dislike doctors who are not up to par. They know the gynecologists who practice sound medicine and those who merely dabble in that specialty. And they are more than aware of doctors who take the stance "Me God, and you idiot." You can't be a nurse without knowing what goes on within the walls of a hospital.

Nurses have one thing going for them. They're not hard to find. You can locate one just by using your head. The building superintendent may tell you there's one in the same apartment house. Or there is probably someone at work who can direct you to one. Or even the next-door neighbor may know one. Don't take her advice about a doctor, but she is as good as anyone to get you to a nurse. Give the nurse a call and tell her you are new in town and that you need a gynecologist. Most general-duty nurses will be courteous and pleased to give you their opinion. Even if the nurse is not personally involved in surgery, the hospital grapevine will have told her who the best surgeon is.

Do nurses have their favorites? Will you get biased opinions from them? Well, nearly everything we get these days has some bias attached to it. Nurses are no exception. Maybe the nurse will send you to the gynecologist who for whatever reason is a favorite of hers. But one thing is certain. She will never send you to the gynecologist who should never have gone into surgery. And you will never end up with one of those general practitioner–surgeons who is skating on thin ice whenever he picks up the scalpel.

Nurses are not the only source of "insider information," even for women living in large metropolitan areas. For instance, an X-ray or laboratory technician, a medical record-room worker, a medical secretary, or even the hospital's maintenance engineer—all have access to the hospital grapevine and can find out for you who is a capable gynecologist. And I think it is worthwhile to mention one other source for women who move to a smaller community and who quickly need the name of the best gynecologist in the area. Try calling the hospital's switchboard operator. She usually knows who's who in the gynecology department. You can't plug in telephones day after day without being tuned into who the best surgeons are. If you want to ask her opinion, remember to call her late in the evening when she's bored. Sometimes she has been instructed to give you a list of the doctors. But if you play your cards right, ten to one says that she will eventually give her opinion on who she would want to do her own hysterectomy. I'd bet on her rather than on those Yellow Pages in the telephone book.

Suppose you already have a family doctor and need a hysterectomy? You may want to put your complete confidence in his opinion of what surgeon you should go to. But there is one catch. He may not want to give it to you. He, too, may hand you a list of a few surgeons. Some doctors believe it's a more democratic approach. They don't want to send all their work to one gynecologist. Others want to hedge on the risk. If something goes wrong, you made the final choice. But it may be that your newness in a community does not give you total trust in his advice. Or you may want to do some digging yourself. It may be the only operation you will ever have. Why not do a little thinking about it yourself?

Are there any other ways to find a competent gynecologist?

This is a long shot, but the one person who has a ring-side seat day after day is the surgical scrub-nurse. She knows the insecure diddlers from the adept surgeons. The ones that sponge out the uterus in two or three hours and the ones that do it with class in an hour. They may hate some gynecologists for their prima donna attitude, but if they are good, they will give credit where it's due. Forget all the other advice I've given you if you are lucky enough to get the name of a scrub-nurse.

What would a doctor do if he moved to a new city and his wife required a hysterectomy? He would call up the hospital and ask to speak to one of the anesthetists. He would ask him a very simple question: "Who would you have to carry out a hysterectomy on your wife?" He would follow his advice without any question. The anesthetist, like the scrub-nurse, is close to where everything is happening. He sees different surgeons in all types of situations. The anesthetist has one other asset. He is not dependent on the surgeon for referrals and will therefore give you an unbiased opinion on the best gynecologist in town. You would be well advised to ask his opinion if you happen to know one.

Having found your gynecologist, don't listen to any gossip about him. If you find out at the last minute that he's an inveterate gambler or has an unpleasant personality, don't rush to cancel the operation. Remember, it's not the morality or the personality that makes the incision.

ARE ALL MALE GYNECOLOGISTS "CHAUVINISTS"?

This topic has to be discussed in a book dealing with hysterectomy. Most gynecologists are males. This situation will change in the years ahead, but right now, it's a fact. And there is no doubt we have been placed squarely on the firing line by a number of angry women's groups. There is also little doubt that some gynecologists are chauvinists and that they, like some other gynecologists, add to the list of needless hysterectomies. But, unlike these other doctors, they cause their patients many additional problems. This section will show you how to handle a chauvinistic gynecologist, but it will also point out that, in some instances possibly "The lady doth protest too much."

Although it's apparent that many women are happy with the medical care they receive from their doctors, an increasing number resent their paternalistic attitude. This is particularly offensive today when the general public is well aware that not all doctors are paragons of virtue. Quite the contrary. But even if this were not the case, more and more women want complete control over their own bodies. Yet many doctors fail to hear this message, continuing to act as "benevolent monarchs" to their patients.

Women's organizations are therefore quite justified in arguing that in certain areas the male-dominated specialty of gynecology is responsible for much personal and social injustice. Some gynecologists will have nothing to do with contraception. The teenager who finally gets up sufficient nerve to ask for the pill may receive a stern lecture on morality instead of walking away with the prescription. It's a bad introduction to the medical profession, and some girls never forget it. Other gynecologists similarly condemn sterilization and abortion. I'm sure that most women would concur that it is a doctor's religious and moral right to steer away from these issues if he wishes to do so. But surely it is also his duty to refer such patients to other gynecologists with more liberal views. Regrettably, some doctors won't even go to that trouble. It can be even more upsetting when these same physicians go to great lengths to undermine these procedures. And it's the final straw when some of these custodians of morality have one standard of behavior for their patients and another for their own families. I received a good deal of criticism on one occasion when I suggested that a well-trained chimpanzee with a stethoscope around his neck would deal more justly with these controversial issues than most doctors do.

Women may also have good reason to complain about the general treatment they receive in the gynecologist's office. Some doctors are rough and approach the woman as if she were a bag of potatoes. One woman gynecologist recently made the point extremely well in the *Annals of Internal Medicine.* She suggested that the way to ensure that male doctors would not perform rough pelvic examinations lay in their training in medical school. Place the male students in stirrups, she advised, and have a strange female doctor come into the room, "squeeze their balls, and leave without saying a word!" There's no doubt this would leave a lasting impression, and it could well be the answer for inconsiderate doctors. The pelvic examination is a very personal and sensitive matter, and should be approached with gentleness and courtesy, along with an adequate explanation.

But is there a sinister chauvinistic plot to subject women to needless hysterectomies? It is over this issue that some women's liberation groups may be reading too much into the script. On the surface a plot might appear to be the case. As I mentioned earlier, more hysterectomies are performed on American women than on women in England or Sweden. But American males also have more surgery than men in other countries. For example, American men have twice the chance of having their hemorrhoids removed as do Englishmen. Canadian men have two and one-half times the chance of undergoing a prostatectomy operation as do Englishmen, and they also face a greater number of vein-stripping procedures, appendectomies, and gallbladder operations. One congressional subcommittee report estimated that 29 percent of the prostatectomies and 22 percent of the hysterectomies performed in the United States could not be medically justified. If there is a sinister master plot to wheel American women into the operating room, it would appear to also include U.S. males.

I have been involved in gynecology too long not to realize that for years women have been subjected to a "moralistic stratagem" by unthinking and arrogant doctors, some of them women doctors. Time and time again I have seen it cause patients untold personal suffering. It is also because of my views on abortion, along with practicing what I preached, that I've been picketed for months at a time by antiabortionists, and been exposed to their lies and abuse. Moreover, in my desire to liberalize abortion at my hospital, I am also quite cognizant of who gave me the most trouble. It wasn't the Roman Catholic clergy or their congregations or even the pickets. It was my own colleagues who continually threw up more roadblocks than James Bond could ever dream up. But although I've frequently condemned these doctors for their unswerving philosophical views, I cannot honestly accuse them of any sinister, overt intrigue to "hysterectomize" women. There are too many other ways to remove the uterus without having to resort to this means.

It is also interesting to speculate on how valid are the psychiatrists' explanations for the increased pelvic surgery. In their opinion women tend to look on the doctor as a figure of authority. It's therefore easy, they say, for susceptible women to slide into a childlike, dependent role with their surgeon. There is some logic to this theory, particularly if the gynecologist has also delivered their children. Having a baby is a very special moment. It rightfully leaves most women with a feeling of great admiration for their doctor. Possibly on this basis one can concede a point or two to the psychiatrists. But patients of both sexes can become extremely dependent on their physician and, when stricken with a serious disease, accept his word as gospel. I've seen many of my colleagues fall under the same kind of spell. Let them develop an illness and they will give you a blow-by-blow analysis of what their doctor has suggested to them. There's a good argument, therefore, for saying it's the patient's personality, rather than anything else, that is the overriding factor in how he or she regards the doctor.

How should women handle a male gynecologist who assumes a strong chauvinistic stance toward them? There is only one way. Change doctors and get the treatment you want, both psychologically and physically. It is useless to believe that you can change the gynecologist's attitude. Besides, it's not your job to do so. Physicians who have not early learned the ABC's of politeness and good manners are never going to acquire them.

It is also advisable to cut your losses early. The wise investor quickly sells a poor stock and licks his wounds. You should use the same approach with doctors. Don't allow the decision to drag into months or even years before you finally decide to make your move. The gynecologist who handles you roughly with the speculum may be even worse when a serious decision is involved. Don't get caught in this trap. You should establish good rapport with a gynecologist long before a hysterectomy or other major problem arises.

6
The
"Knick-Nack-Ectomy"

Initially this may appear to be an odd term in a book dealing with hysterectomy, yet it's not meant to be flippant or frivolous. Rather it should be considered a very important matter, since the "knick-nack-ectomy" operation often causes women more harm than a questionable hysterectomy.

A "knick-nack-ectomy" is anything short of a hysterectomy. The following case is hypothetical, but it could well be true. It is a prime example of how a patient can repeatedly be led astray, not only by the family doctor, but also by a well-qualified specialist.

It started when Florence G. was eighteen years of age. During the night she was awakened by an acute pain in her right side. Her mother hurriedly called the family doctor, telling him she thought it was an attack of appendicitis because the symptoms were the same as those her younger daughter had had two years earlier when she had been rushed to the hospital for an operation. The doctor agreed that it was appendicitis, and since the diagnosis appeared obvious to everyone, neither the family nor the doctor suggested a consultation. Dr. X had been given operating privileges at the hospital for a number of so-called minor procedures, and later that night he did a good job in removing the appendix. There was only one problem—it was a normal appendix.

Florence arrived home toward the end of the week, and her parents were pleased that there were no complications. But Dr. X. never explained the exact circumstances of the case. Why should he have? The parents were satisfied with his care. Yet, in retrospect, he had made a hasty move. In the rush to get to the operating room, he had been sloppy in neglecting to ask Florence some questions about her periods. It would have been logical to inquire if the pain had started halfway between periods. The hard truth was that she had ruptured a small cyst at the time of ovulation. Some women may be aware of a small amount of pain each month when ovulation occurs. But on rare occasions it can be severe for a few hours and simulate an attack of appendicitis if the cyst is on the right side. Doctors call this condition "Mittelschmerz," or "middle pain," and observing the patient for a short time will usually prevent a needless appendectomy.

When Florence was twenty-five, during her annual appointment for a Pap cancer smear, her doctor felt an orange-sized ovarian cyst to the left side of the uterus. He told her it should be removed, and once again he opened her abdomen. This was a greater error than the first operation. Florence was young. She was not in pain. And besides, she didn't need an incision. The doctor should have been less trigger-happy with the scalpel. If he had waited and done a repeat pelvic examination in six weeks, the cyst probably would have been gone. Orange-sized cysts in young girls frequently disappear on their own with no treatment. But it was the same old routine—a quick operation and no thought of calling in a consultant. Now, at twenty-five, Florence had two scars and had lost a normal ovary.

The next year Florence married, and soon had two children. Following her second pregnancy she developed painful periods and a nagging pain in her left side. Her doctor diagnosed the problem as an infection of her left tube and suggested its removal. So at age thirty she had her third operation, to excise the tube. The pathology reported it as a normal tube, but Florence never heard about this finding.

It was at this point that Florence and her family moved to another city. She continued to have occasional bouts of pain in her left side, and she had begun to suffer from painful intercourse, which was soon causing some marital strife. She was now thirty-six and was told by her new doctor that she had a tipped uterus. The diagnosis was correct. Most tipped wombs are of no significance, but this one had been firmly pulled back by adhesions from her previous operations. It was now adherent to the end of the vagina and was repeatedly struck during intercourse. The doctor's advice was to have an operation to suspend the uterus.

Florence and her husband didn't rush into this decision. They first asked if a hysterectomy could be done. It was not their intention to have another child. Wouldn't it be better to go all the way this time? But their family doctor argued against it. He said she was too young. Little did they know that there was another reason he recommended a uterine suspension rather than a hysterectomy. He, too, was a general practitioner–surgeon, but he had never been given operating privileges to perform hysterectomies. It would mean referring the patient to a gynecologist if a more major operation were to be done. A couple of days prior to her thirty-sixth birthday, Florence's uterus was suspended, and, fortunately, this did relieve the pain during intercourse.

Four years later Florence began to notice an increase in her menstrual flow. Several months went by, and then she suddenly hemorrhaged, the bleeding continuing for three weeks. This time she was referred to a gynecologist and was told that a large fibroid was present. A hysterectomy was the only sensible treatment. Florence readily consented to the operation, believing that this fifth operation would finally end her pelvic problems. The gynecologist assured her this was the case, and the operation was performed. At age forty it now looked as though all her troubles were past history.

During the next ten years Florence's health had never been better. Then, during her fiftieth year, she slowly became aware that she was gradually putting on weight. Her clothes seemed tight around her abdomen, and she had a constant bloating sensation. It was only when she began to notice pain that she reluctantly made an appointment to see the gynecologist. He told her she had a large cystic mass in the pelvic cavity and admitted it could be a cancer. At the time of hysterectomy he had decided to leave in her right ovary. This had kept Florence from starting the menopause, but that ovary was now the size of a small football. Florence was lucky. It was a benign, noncancerous cyst. It was also her sixth operation.

HOW TO PREVENT
BECOMING A "PELVIC CRIPPLE"

Florence is a typical example of the patient who has too many "knick-nack-ectomies." She had been subjected to six operations, yet only one of these was necessary. A single total hysterectomy at age forty should have been her only incision. How could she have prevented what happened to her?

Her family made the first error by not insisting on a consultation before the appendectomy was performed. This mistake was compounded with each incision. Florence ended up with a checkerboard abdomen, full of scars. But, more important, these operations produced an increasing amount of adhesions in the pelvic cavity. This is what eventually makes a woman a "pelvic cripple." The scar tissue takes the normal mobility out of the pelvic structures. Usually the uterus can move back and forward in the pelvis. The scar tissue removes this elasticity and also pulls the organs into fixed, abnormal positions. The greater the number of operations, the greater the chances this will happen and pelvic pain will result.

At the point where Florence's doctor recommended a uterine suspension, Florence herself should have used common sense. She and her husband did momentarily question this operation when they wondered if a hysterectomy should be done. It was a logical question. She had no desire for another child. This would be her fourth operation. Why not make it a final, definitive hysterectomy? Unfortunately, they gave in too easily to their doctor's advice and did not insist on another opinion.

Florence's gynecologist also used poor judgment. He

was recommending a necessary fifth operation. Why leave in an old ovary and risk the chance of still another operation? Even if Florence were having her first operation, it would have been a questionable move. A well-informed and thinking patient could have prevented further trouble by realizing that there was a choice of either leaving the ovary in or taking it out. Most people at this juncture would tell the surgeon to end any possibility of future operations. He could easily have excised the remaining ovary and placed Florence on a daily estrogen pill to prevent the start of the menopause. We will talk more about this in Chapter 11.

In the practice of gynecology the occasional "knick-nack-ectomy" is a "must" operation. For instance, if an ovarian cyst persists in a young girl, it should be removed. Similarly, a badly tipped uterus in a newly married woman that is causing severe pain during intercourse may require a suspension procedure. It would be totally irresponsible to carry out a hysterectomy under these circumstances. The "knick-nack-ectomy" is therefore indicated if there is a sound reason for the operation and the timing is right. But the repetitive removal of parts of the female organs by general practitioners who dabble in surgery is not giving American women a fair deal. It is sexual inequality at its worst. Make certain it doesn't happen to you.

7
D and C or Hysterectomy?

Some doctors never give their patients any control or choice in their own treatment. But there are situations in gynecology when the most chauvinistic surgeon will suddenly place his female patient on the horns of a dilemma by asking her whether she prefers to enter the hospital for a D and C or a hysterectomy. Sometimes the question is posed merely to gauge the patient's reaction to a hysterectomy. If she quickly backs away from it, so will the surgeon. But if she eagerly reaches for the operation, the doctor knows he's on safe ground and may push harder in that direction.

Yet some surgeons are completely sincere when they ask the question. Their purpose is to quickly assess which procedure is more psychologically acceptable to the patient. They know, from adding up the medical facts, that a situation such as abnormal bleeding can be handled either way, and it makes little difference which way the pendulum swings. In effect, they have room to maneuver. This should not be looked on by patients as anything bad. Yet I've seen innumerable women confused and worried when confronted with a choice.

When the gynecologist gives a woman this option, he is first of all, in essence, telling her that he doesn't think a cancer is present. Patients with a definite malignancy are never handed this kind of choice. If the woman's problem is abnormal bleeding, a D and C may help or cure it, but the point is that it also may not help—the bleeding may not be controlled, and a hysterectomy will eventually be required. If the doctor has made the decision and this happens—a hysterectomy is necessary after all—and the patient is then told she has to go back into the hospital, she may blame the doctor. She reasons, "Why didn't he do a hysterectomy the first time?" Obviously, she doesn't care that for other women the doctor's choice of a D and C was the right one. She knows only that it turned out to be the wrong move for her. She also invariably forgets that hindsight is much easier than foresight. The doctor therefore says to himself, "Let the patient make the final decision on this one, just in case she blames me later on."

Patients have another problem when they are suddenly given a choice. The doctor fails to provide sufficient information for them to weigh the pros and cons of each approach. It may be just because the doctor is pressed for time, or he may assume the patient knows more than she does about the problem. Or he may be one of those physicians who have never had the ability to explain medical troubles in an easy fashion. But even if the doctor has done a creditable job of explanation, the patient's tension may fog the issue. Once home, all the pros and cons become a total blank. Hopefully, knowing about some common problems ahead of time will help steer you in the right direction. The following examples illustrate that in the surgical game there are times when it's advisable to be very conservative and on other occasions it is wiser to accept a more radical route to solve the problem. Much depends on what has happened in the past, the diagnosis, your age, and whether or not there is any desire for a future pregnancy.

Let's first discuss what could be best described as the "D and C syndrome." Every gynecologist sees women in their thirties and forties who have undergone five or six D and C's. The usual story is a long, stormy history of abnormal bleeding—frequent and heavy periods, prolonged periods, or very irregular episodes of bleeding when there appears to be no rhyme or reason to the menstrual pattern. One quickly gets the impression that these women have had one problem after another since the start of their periods. This constant annoyance has resulted in a D and C every year or two, which temporarily decreases, but never solves, the problem. In looking back over these repetitive procedures, it is impossible for a new doctor to know how many of them were necessary. Yet he has the feeling that it has become somewhat of a habit. Moreover, if he takes the time to gather up all the past reports from the pathologist, in the great majority of cases the tissue will always have been normal. This does not necessarily imply the D and C's were not justified, but it does mean that someone should have used a little more common sense and called a halt at an earlier date.

Gynecologists refer to this problem as "dysfunctional bleeding," which was discussed in Chapter 2. It means that doctors cannot lay their fingers on any disease, and in one sense, therefore, it is a good diagnosis, giving the gyne-

cologist three avenues of treatment. If a woman has already undergone five D and C's, one might wonder why
any doctor would suggest another one. In select cases, in
spite of what I've said earlier, it does make sense. For instance, if she is very near the menopause, maybe one
more will control the bleeding long enough to tide her
over. And if she hasn't had a D and C for a few years,
some problem may have developed in the interim. Another D and C will rule out the chance that "dysfunctional
bleeding" has changed into "disease bleeding." So don't
shy away from another D and C if you happen to be in this
group of patients.

The doctor may say, however, that he wants to try the
birth-control pill for a few months to determine if this will
hold the periods in check. Similarly, it might control the
bleeding just long enough to enable the patient to reach
the menopause. But before putting her on the pill, he will
insist on a D and C, if she hasn't had one for several years,
to preclude the possibility of a malignancy.

But if the woman is in her thirties or forties, with five
D and C's behind her and no desire for a future pregnancy, it makes no sense to continue playing this losing
game. A hysterectomy is the only reasonable route to get
rid of the "D and C syndrome."

Now let's see how the diagnosis may affect the decision. Some women, following a D and C, will be told that
they have endometrial hyperplasia, the condition where
the lining of the uterus is thicker than normal and heavier
bleeding occurs. (This, too, is discussed in Chapter 2.) Fortunately, this problem may sometimes be cured by that
single D and C. But if bleeding recurs, it becomes questionable whether further D and C's should be done. Hyperplasia can be a progressive condition, and in some in-

stances it may change into a malignancy. Removing the uterus prevents this potential hazard. If a doctor suggests a hysterectomy under these circumstances, it makes sense to follow that advice.

In general it's not a good idea to procrastinate with definite disease. This does not imply that if a small fibroid is detected during a routine checkup, it should quickly be removed. Let's assume that a gynecologist has performed a D and C because of heavy and prolonged periods. He later informs the patient that a small fibroid is present in the wall of the uterus and that it might result in further episodes of profuse bleeding. Under these circumstances it is still better to play a "wait-and-see" game. The patient may be lucky, particularly if she is a few months away from the menopause. But if the bleeding again becomes a problem, additional D and C's are a waste of time. She is usually merely putting off the inevitable. Furthermore, she is exposing herself to the potential dangers of another anesthetic. This is the time to have a "needed hysterectomy."

The D and C, like the hysterectomy, is often a questionable procedure, but it is much harder to police its abuses. It can be a life saving operation when it picks up an early cancer of the uterus. Yet frequently it is sold to the patient for "gray-area" reasons. The best that women can do is to shy away from the "D and C syndrome." If you are having this procedure every year or two, be sure to ask for a consultation before the next one.

8
What You Should Know Before the Hysterectomy

IS OBESITY OF IMPORTANCE?

Many obese women will need a hysterectomy this year and will be advised to lose weight before the operation. How forcefully the patients are told to do so usually depends on the age of the surgeon. A young gynecologist will tell them with great conviction to lose the excess poundage. But an older doctor may do it in a rather half-hearted way. You really can't blame the more mature surgeon for taking a softer stand on obesity. He has gone through the routine so frequently and failed so often that psychologically he long ago gave up the battle of the bulge. I am therefore under no illusion that what I have to say here will have much, if any, effect on decreasing obesity prior to surgery. But it will at least document the importance of "surgical obesity."

It's a well-publicized fact that obesity is more than a

cosmetic problem. Life insurance companies have repeatedly stessed that overweight policyholders have a shorter life expectancy than lean ones. The cold, blunt, unalterable fact is that obese patients of both sexes are more prone to flat feet, diabetes, hypertension, arthritis, and a host of other problems. We also know that obese women are more likely to develop menstrual troubles, thyroid dysfunction, and cancer of the uterus. In fact, nearly half of the patients with uterine cancer are clearly obese.

What isn't well publicized is that obesity is a major surgical hazard. The casual onlooker might conclude it would be twice as hard to perform a hysterectomy on a 250-pound woman as on a 125-pound woman. But it actually is many times more difficult for the gynecologist, particularly one who isn't overly adept under the best of circumstances. It takes a skilled technical surgeon, using all the tricks he's learned, to safely carry out a hysterectomy on an obese woman.

It's not just the surgeon who has problems with an overweight patient. The anesthetist also has his problems. It may be difficult to find a good vein to start the intravenous drip, or to intubate so as to ensure an adequate supply of gases into the lungs. It becomes a fight for all the doctors from the beginning to the end of the operation. And following the surgery obese patients simply don't have that tiger in the tank that helps to get thin patients moving. Furthermore, in general, obese women have more postoperative complications, such as wound infections, disruption of the incision, phlebitis, or pneumonia.

At the moment, no one has found a way to get this vital message through to hysterectomy patients. Sometimes there isn't sufficient time to lose weight. But even if there is, diets, health clubs, and all the pleadings from the gynecologist rarely bring results. I've often pondered if a "money approach" would work. For centuries surgeons have charged by the patient. What if they suddenly decided to bill patients by the pound? Would that finally get the message across that obesity is a grave peril for either sex? It might save a few lives. And it would certainly help to relieve the coronary spasm many surgeons feel when they contemplate operating on an obese patient.

AM I TOO OLD?

While I was writing this book, her family doctor asked me to see Esther J., a charming eighty-three-year-old woman who still had the ability and zest for living life to the fullest extent. For the last year she had been forced to curtail some of her activities because she found it impossible to control her urine. The embarrassment of continually getting up from a wet chair finally forced her to give up going out.

Now Esther was in my office asking what could be done to correct it. It was no use telling her that she was too old. Initially, her general practitioner had used this argument, but she had refused to accept it as a valid excuse. He was then prompted to ask a cardiologist to give her a thorough workup. He concluded, following a series of tests, that she was in excellent shape for her age and should be seen by a gynecologist.

This alert, sprightly woman was a prime example of chronological versus biological age. She may have been eighty-three, but she got on and off the examining table with the nimbleness of a woman twenty years her junior.

She came from solid, long-living stock, and her parts were not wearing out as quickly as other women's. Her mother had lived to be ninety-four, and her father to be eighty-nine. There was every reason to suspect that Esther would equal or better their records.

The pelvic examination revealed a falling-down of the uterus and bladder, and the only good treatment was surgery. But should an eighty-three-year-old woman be exposed to a major operation? It's a question many elderly patients or their families ask the doctor. Children who love their aging parents genuinely worry that they are simply too old to be subjected to the trauma of surgery. It's an understandable concern, and one that will be more and more in the minds of American families. People are living longer, and, as happens with an aging car, an increasing number of wear-and-tear problems will become surgical problems for them.

It is impossible to generalize too much about patients in their seventies and eighties, but over the years I've formed some basic opinions about them. One is that old people are tough and usually do amazingly well after surgery. Maybe it's in part because at their age they have developed a mature philosophy of life. But I think the primary reason is they already have a proven track record of health to have survived as long as they have. Right from the moment of conception the genes were the correct ones for a long and healthy life.

But although time and time again I've seen elderly women scramble out of bed earlier than much younger patients, it's imperative to handle them with extra care. By this age every person has developed some chronic problem that may add an additional hazard to the operation. For instance, chronic chest trouble may change into a postoperative pneumonia. It's important, therefore, to cure the anemia, or make certain the diabetes, hypertension, or any other abnormality is as well controlled as possible prior to embarking on a major operation.

Esther eventually had a hysterectomy along with repair of her bladder. She was home in ten days and back to her activities six weeks later. Hopefully, she will live another ten years or more, but regardless of how long, she was now able to live rather than merely exist. In the opinion of many doctors, this is one of the primary reasons for deciding to proceed with surgery with patients in this age group. Obviously, everyone has to assume an additional risk at this time of life. But that should in no way preclude an operation if it can be justified and the patient is in reasonable health.

HOW MANY PROBLEMS ❀ WILL THE HYSTERECTOMY CURE?

Women who are realistic and practical will normally experience good results from a hysterectomy. They are not seeking miracles, merely relief from bona fide complaints. On the other hand, women who expect the operation to cure all the aches and pains in their bodies and also solve a multitude of long-term emotional problems, are in for disappointment. They have set their sights too high or have simply aimed at the wrong goals. It is these women who frequently condemn the operation because it has failed to live up to their unreasonable expectations. Knowing beforehand what a hysterectomy will and will not do can prevent this disappointment.

What are the sure things about a hysterectomy? First,

obviously, women cannot become pregnant following the operation. Second, it removes both menstruation and menstrual pain. Third, it eliminates the chance of uterine cancer. But there the certainty stops and "gray-area" results come into play.

What about abdominal pain or discomfort during intercourse? Will these symptoms be relieved by a hysterectomy? The answer depends primarily on the diagnosis and the reason for the operation. For example, if the abdominal pain results from a huge fibroid uterus or a severe pelvic infection, the outcome should be rewarding. Similarly, if there has been extensive endometriosis, or internal bleeding, which has caused scarring of the ligaments at the end of the vagina, again the symptoms should be relieved. It's logical to assume that cutting away the disease usually solves the problem. If, however, at the time of surgery there's nothing significant to excise, the patient's hopes for relief from a variety of symptoms will not be realized. And postoperative psychological and emotional pangs may haunt both patient and surgeon.

It should always be remembered that pelvic complaints may have a multifocal origin. After all, very few things in life are 100 percent situations. For instance, part of a backache may be due to a large fibroid. But another part of it may result from a lumbosacral strain. And both these troubles can be aggravated by a myriad of personal problems. You cannot excise all of these causes by a hysterectomy. Moreover, regardless of how thorough the surgeon's questions are prior to the operation, it's impossible to estimate how much pain is caused by each condition.

Besides, surgery sometimes provides only temporary

relief from an annoyance. Urinary incontinence from a prolapse of the uterus and bladder, for example, may be totally abated following the operation. But six months later it may have recurred. This type of surgery never comes with definite guarantees, although, fortunately, the long-term results are good in the majority of cases.

Hysterectomy, like any surgical procedure, gives satisfactory results if all the ground rules have been well worked out in advance of the operation. But anyone rushing into it with illogical preconceived ideas, and thinking it is the answer to every prayer, is destined for disappointment.

Does a hysterectomy renew a woman's energy?
This is one of those unreasonable expectations. It would only accomplish this if a woman were suffering from chronic anemia secondary to heavy periods. Putting a stop to this blood loss month after month and prescribing iron to restore the blood to normal could renew her old vigor.

IS THE HYSTERECTOMY A MINOR OPERATION?

Sometimes I hear women say, "I'm just going in for a hysterectomy," implying it's a rather simple, matter-of-fact procedure. Or they'll try to put words in the surgeon's mouth by asking, "I guess it's not much of an operation these days, is it, Doctor?"

Let me quickly set the record straight by telling you about a former professor of surgery at the Harvard Medical School, who once told his students, "There is no such thing as minor surgery, but there are a lot of minor surgeons." This statement is as true today as it was at that time. Hysterectomy should never be looked on as a minor procedure, when thousands of women die because of it.

You merely have to look at the record to realize that the term "minor surgery" is a misnomer. A patient was admitted to the hospital for removal of an ingrown toenail and died because of reaction to the anesthetic; an eight-month-old baby succumbed from a circumcision operation; a healthy twenty-two-year-old woman had a cardiac arrest immediately after a D and C. Of course, these are rare occurrences, but if they do strike the patient, they are direct hits, and it would be impossible to convince the families of such patients that these were minor procedures. No matter how routine the procedure, there is always an element of risk.

There is no doubt that present-day surgeons have an excellent batting average compared to those in earlier years. But this is the very thing that is deceptive. It's become routine to see women enter the hospital and, in the great majority of cases, shortly be discharged without problems. But another surgeon, recalling some trying moments in his long surgical career, said, "Surgery is like flying—ninety-nine percent boredom and one percent sheer terror." Every seasoned surgeon can recall with horror occasions in the operating room when a patient's life hung in the balance.

The hysterectomy operation has become an exceedingly safe procedure if the right surgeon is performing it. But never make the mistake of classifying it as a minor procedure. Too often, this approach opens the door to needless hysterectomies.

DON'T PUSH YOURSELF
INTO THE WRONG TIME SLOT

It's been aptly said that part of one's success in life depends on being the right person in the right place at the right time. This philosophy also applies to the hysterectomy operation. Some women, for instance, without realizing it, increase the risk of surgery by being in the wrong time slot, although in certain cases they have no control over it.

In *Wheels,* novelist Arthur Hailey cautioned about buying cars that were built on Mondays and Fridays. Monday's cars, he said, may have some of the weekend hangover built into them. And Friday's cars sometimes lack the nuts and bolts left out by a worker who wants to get away for a fishing trip. It would take a sophisticated computer to ascertain how much "Hailey's Law" applies to the hysterectomy. But there's reason to suspect the computer would find that there are some days better than others on which to have a hysterectomy. And I doubt that it would choose either Monday or Friday to have its own nuts and bolts tightened up.

Surgeons are not mechanical robots, and now and then they unwittingly fall into bad habits. For example, the most skillful and dedicated surgeon in the hospital may routinely arrive home from his weekend cottage on Sundays at midnight, and he's not quite as sharp for his 8:00 A.M. Monday case as he will be the following day. Similarly, on Friday he's had a full, tiring week. You can't expect him to be as sharp as he was earlier in the week. And possibly there's an element of rush to Friday's operation. He has a full morning of surgery. It's also going to be a tight squeeze getting through a full quota of afternoon patients. Besides, he told his wife he would try to get away earlier this weekend.

Most surgeons would therefore pick Tuesday at 8:00 A.M. if they had to have an operation themselves. The Monday-morning cobwebs are gone. And in the event of a complication during the day or two following the operation, the surgeon will be readily available. Also, you can't beat 8:00 A.M. as the time to be wheeled into the operating room. The surgeon, anesthetist, and nurses are all fresh. I'm sure the computer would be able to plot a gradual decrease in everyone's efficiency with each succeeding case. There is also one other important point about the 8:00 A.M. operation. It always starts on time. The ones that follow it rarely do. The earlier surgeons take longer than their allotted time, and everyone else becomes a late starter. The ground, therefore, becomes ripe for surgeons to try to make up a little lost time. And as the old adage warns, "The more haste, the less speed." Clock watching is a poor way to play the surgical game.

There's another time pitfall. Let's assume you've been in the hospital for several days, undergoing treatment for some gynecological problem. The doctor finally decides that a hysterectomy should be done, but there is no urgency about it. It would be a normal reaction to want it performed while you are still in the hospital. But remember that occupying a bed does not automatically give you operating time—unless it is an emergency. Elective surgery is scheduled many weeks in advance. If your operation could be scheduled, it might mean having it done at 5:00 P.M., at the end of the OR list. It would also mean that a tired surgeon had to return to the hospital after a long afternoon of office hours. Don't play the game that way. You would be well advised to go home and to ask the surgeon for that Tuesday morning at 8:00 A.M.

Not everyone can insist on 8:00 A.M. Tuesday for an operation. Maybe a surgeon can, but what about the person on the street?

It may be a problem to get the prime time slot, but why not at least ask the surgeon for that time? You have nothing to lose. A "thinking doctor" would try for a top time. What is good for the doctor is equally good for you.

Is there a best time of the year to have a hysterectomy?

It is preferable to shy away from the summer months. The hospital may not have air conditioning, and you might hit a heat wave. You don't want to be fighting the heat as well as the postoperative pain. Operating rooms in the newer hospitals in the United States are always temperature-controlled, but it isn't unusual for air conditioning to break down just when you need it the most. Surgeons are not at their best in 90-degree temperatures. The top gynecologists are also able to take longer vacations than the lesser ones. You could end up with second best if you push for the summer months.

WHY NOT HAVE THE MOLE REMOVED AT THE SAME TIME?

Women who are scheduled for a hysterectomy may at the last minute ask their gynecologists to add something else onto the operation. They may have a mole, an ingrown toenail, a cyst, or even hemorrhoids that they want to get rid of at the same time. After all, they are being put to sleep, so why not kill two birds with one stone?

Some patients bring up the matter just as they are about to enter the OR. If you happen to have something like this on your mind, don't be surprised if the gynecologist quickly turns down the request. Your desire to have a little extra added to the operation is easier said than done. It adds to the operating time, and surgeons don't like disrupting the schedule. In general, most surgeons take longer to do an operation than the time given to them. Adding that "little extra," even if it's just a mole, means shifting the patient's position, another prep of the skin, new instruments. A small cyst on the back could easily put another half hour onto the operating time. A surgeon who steps out of the OR late is holding up everyone else. It's not polite. It also makes him look as if he is losing his touch. Surgeons don't like giving that impression, regardless of whether it's right or wrong. Often a surgeon will say, "Sorry you've been held up, Mike, but it wasn't my fault. I got started late. I hear Bill got into some trouble." In short, "Don't blame me. I'm not losing the old touch."

In the event you want something else done, be sure to ask the surgeon about it at the time he books you for the hysterectomy. He can quickly tell you if it's a wise move. If it is reasonable, everyone, including the OR staff, will be prepared for it.

DON'T GET PREGNANT BEFORE THE HYSTERECTOMY

Some women get very careless about contraception while waiting for a hysterectomy to be done. They seem to adopt the philosophy "Why should I worry about pregnancy when my uterus is going to be removed in a couple of months?" This can be a dangerous attitude that can result in a tremendous amount of grief for the patient. It may also cause a good deal of embarrassment for the surgeon.

Sally B. at age thirty-five had worried about an unwanted pregnancy for the past five years. With four children and an unhappy marriage, she welcomed the hysterectomy recommended for a dropped uterus. Sally was extremely conscientious about always using a contraceptive cream prior to intercourse. Yet, knowing her hysterectomy was a mere six weeks away, she became lax in using it.

A week before the surgery, she developed a severe vaginal irritation, and a pelvic examination diagnosed a fungus infection. It also showed she had an early pregnancy. Sally was a staunch Roman Catholic, but because of bad varicose veins had consented to use a vaginal contraceptive. But when her doctor suggested an abortion, her religious background could not allow her this ultimate means of contraception control. Sally was forced to have a fifth child, complicated by toxemia of pregnancy, and spent two months in the hospital.

Sally B. ended up with an unwanted child. But it could have been worse. Consider the case of Isobel C., a trim, forty-four-year-old woman with three children, the youngest fifteen years of age. She had been on the pill for ten years and was looking forward to being a grandmother. She had been told she had a large, grapefruit-sized fibroid and that a hysterectomy was the only sensible approach. Isobel had also begun to suffer from migraine headaches, and both she and her doctor laid the blame on the pill. "You may as well stop the pill, Isobel," was the doctor's final advice to her as she was leaving the office. But neither party made any mention of some alternate means of contraception. It was an easy trap to fall into, even for the doctor. After all, she was forty-four and also had a large fibroid. Neither of these facts was conducive to a pregnancy.

Isobel's surgery had been put off for three months. She wanted it done in the fall. When the incision was made, the surgeon found the uterus definitely enlarged from a large number of fibroids. But it looked and felt much softer than a fibroid tumor, which could mean she was pregnant. Whether she was or not was not an easy question to answer. A degenerating fibroid uterus can also become quite soft and simulate an early pregnancy.

If a surgeon goes ahead and removes a pregnant uterus, not only does he look foolish in the eyes of his colleagues, but he could be severely criticized by the tissue committee. And, in addition, the patient could cause trouble if she is morally against abortion. But if he backs off and closes the abdomen and the patient isn't pregnant, you can imagine how inept he appears to the patient. On several occasions over the years I have been hurriedly called to the operating room to give an opinion on whether a uterus was enlarged from a fibroid or a pregnancy. It can be a trying and difficult decision. In Isobel C.'s case, the surgeon finally decided that the most likely possibility was a pregnancy, and he closed the incision.

Later that day, a near-hysterical Isobel heard the news and at first refused to believe it. She thought the doctor must be wrong. When pregnancy tests confirmed the surgeon's diagnosis, Isobel had an abortion and immediately went back on the pill. Three months later, when she had recovered from the earlier incision, a hysterectomy was performed.

All these troubles resulted from "careless contraception." How often this complication arises depends on the type of contraception being used by the patient. Women who have an intrauterine device rarely fall into this trap unless the device is removed too early. Most surgeons would not disturb the loop before the operation. It is usually the patients on the pill or those using a vaginal contraceptive who stop using it too soon.

Contraception should be practiced right up to the time of surgery. And those women who have not used any means of birth control for several years should quickly purchase a vaginal contraceptive cream. It could save considerable misery.

HOW LONG WILL IT TAKE TO RECUPERATE?

Women who are scheduled for a hysterectomy usually have two primary questions in the backs of their minds. First: How long will it take to get back to normal? Second: What can I do after I leave the hospital? One problem is that not all patients want to hear the same answers.

It has been my experience over the years that these questions are posed by two types of women. One group is extremely eager to put the operation behind them and return to living an active life. The other group looks on the postoperative period as a means of escape from normal responsibilities. They want the doctor to tell them it will be many months before they can assume their usual work load. This posture has a direct bearing on how long it takes these patients to recuperate. I've known many women who tried to stretch it into several years.

The majority of patients will leave the hospital within seven to ten days. The watchword on arriving home should be common sense and moderation. Those women who want to move quickly into their normal routines sometimes expect too much at this early date. It's impossible for anyone to get their sea legs back ten days after a major operation. Remember how you feel following the common cold! Small wonder that you wear out early in the day after a hysterectomy. This is therefore the time to put your feet up for a few hours a day and relax with a good book or in front of the TV. And get to bed early. I realize that this is easier said than done when a patient may return to a household of several children and a husband who may not be cooperative. The only solution is to let less important chores slide by in those early weeks. And this is the time to take a harder line with everyone in the family.

Here are some of the common questions about what can and cannot be done that have crossed my desk over the years.

How soon can I take a bath?
Contrary to popular belief, water does not enter the vagina during a bath. You may therefore take either a bath or a shower as soon as you arrive home.

Can I do any housework?
Some patients seem to believe that any activity is bad for them. I even had one woman ask, "Can I lift a coffeepot?" Light activity is never going to cause any trouble. In fact, keeping on the go with minimal chores is good for you. The best way to get a ship into trouble is to keep it in port too long. Just remember to stay away from heavy lifting

and extreme stretching. Obviously you shouldn't decide this is the time to rearrange the furniture or clean the ceiling.

When can I climb stairs?

You can easily go up and down stairs anytime without causing injury to the incision.

When can I return to work?

This depends on your job. Many women feel strong enough to get back to the office in a month's time. The average length of time would be about six weeks. But if your job requires moderate lifting, wait for ten to twelve weeks.

When can I start playing tennis again?

You should wait three months before going back to any active sport.

How soon can I drive a car?

This is always a hard question to answer. In general, it's preferable to delay it for a few weeks. But if you have an automatic gearshift and all the power equipment, you could get behind the wheel in a week or two. But use more than the usual care while driving.

When can I go for a drive with someone else at the wheel?

Anytime.

My husband is leaving on a business trip three weeks after I arrive home. It means driving about six hundred miles. Could I go along?

It's too early for comfort. During the hysterectomy the uterus is cut away from the end of the vagina. It takes this area about six weeks to heal. Most likely you would not get into any trouble, but don't push your luck. The constant jogging of the car might start some bleeding. You would be better advised to stay at home.

How about traveling by air?
My general policy is for patients to stay close to home for six weeks. It is the safest course.

When can I start douching?
Wait until your doctor has done a pelvic examination in six weeks' time.

When can I resume doing exercises?
The same advice applies as for heavy lifting or for active sports. Wait for three months.

Is it necessary to take vitamins or a tonic?
Most women don't need them either prior to or after an operation.

What about sex?
You must wait until the doctor has done a pelvic examination. Generally speaking, it takes anywhere from six to eight weeks for the vaginal incision to heal.

DOES THE TYPE OF HOSPITAL MAKE ANY DIFFERENCE?

I'm often asked if it makes any difference what kind of hospital a woman enters for a hysterectomy. It's a good question and one that more American women should give some thought to. Just as there are good and poor surgeons, so are there high- and low-grade hospitals. If you can end up with both a topflight surgeon and one of the better hospitals, it is obviously the best combination.

In the United States there are over seven thousand hospitals. Of these, around forty-seven hundred are accredited by the Joint Commission on Accreditation of Hospitals (JCAH). The American College of Surgeons instituted the JCAH in 1918 in order to raise the standard of surgical care. Now, however, this organization looks not only at the surgical aspects but also at other departments of the hospital. In effect it attempts to determine whether a particular hospital follows a minimum set of standards. Does the surgical tissue committee function to ensure that the operation was warranted? Do the patients' charts show that they received adequate treatment? Are the hospital administrators up to par? These and many other questions are tabulated to ascertain whether the hospital should be accredited or should be allowed to keep its accredited status.

There is no doubt that the JCAH has helped to raise the general standards of surgical care in the United States. Having "Big Brother" looking over one's shoulder keeps everyone on his toes. But any watchdog association can go only so far in policing the medical profession. It can help to pinpoint and correct gross deficiencies in patient care, but it cannot constantly police a surgeon's conscience. We saw earlier that there are many variables determining whether or not a needless hysterectomy is performed. It's impossible to expect that tissue committees, audits of surgical charts, or anything else the JCAH could institute would adequately police these "gray-area" problems. You always have to return to the more reliable formula—a thinking, informed patient and a doctor you trust.

Does the stamp of approval of the JCAH ensure that all the surgeons in a hospital are well qualified to perform a hysterectomy?

It depends on what is meant by the phrase "well qualified." Accredited hospitals have more surgeons who are members of the American Board of Surgery and the American Board of Obstetrics and Gynecology. But you can't make a silk purse out of a sow's ear. Some surgeons have all the right diplomas hanging on the wall, but they will never be good technical surgeons. I don't know of any organization in either the United States or Canada that really checks out a surgeon's hands. So don't count on the JCAH to ensure this aspect of the surgeon's qualifications. Use the "insider-information" approach that I discussed in Chapter 5.

What if the hospital my doctor is affiliated with isn't accredited?

In general, it is preferable to be in an accredited hospital. But there are many excellent doctors in nonaccredited hospitals. Moreover, some of these hospitals do a creditable job of caring for patients. It is much better to have a first-class surgeon in one of these hospitals than a questionable surgeon in an accredited hospital.

Would going to a large clinic assure one of getting a better surgeon?

If it were a choice between picking a surgeon in your area haphazardly or entering a large clinic and being given a surgeon without knowing who's who in that institution, your chances of hitting a poor surgeon would be smaller at the clinic. Prestigious clinics don't tolerate borderline surgeons. Hospitals have less control. But, once again, if you are willing to do a little legwork and can use the "insider approach" to advantage, there is no need to spend money for faraway clinics.

9
How to Guard Against Emotional Problems Before and After the Hysterectomy

Age-old misconceptions about hysterectomy are remarkably persistent in spite of widening knowledge and more open discussion of the subject. And, surprisingly, new horror stories are gaining credence as a result of feminist skepticism. Both cause needless worry.

Fortunately, the prophets of doom are not making as much headway as in former years. Most women no longer worry that they are going to grow a beard, become obese, or lose their sexual drive following a hysterectomy. They seem to be taking a more reasoned and practical approach, and, once convinced the operation is needed for a bona fide problem, they are eager to rid themselves of annoying, and sometimes incapacitating, symptoms, or are gratified that a precancerous lesion can be completely cured.

It's possible to argue that even the prevalent concern about the "needless hysterectomy" has helped to develop this attitude because any controversy about hysterectomy brings it out into the open. In any case, familiarity with the subject has removed much of the element of fear from the procedure. Women who are preparing for the operation can look at the track record of numerous friends who have emerged from it successfully and are willing to talk about it. The old dictum about safety in numbers has had a salutary effect.

Another reassuring note is that increasing age decreases the chance of emotional distress. For example, those young women who develop a depression following a pregnancy have a high incidence of previous psychiatric disorders. The pregnancy has brought the trouble to the surface. Some authorities believe that about 50 percent of these patients have underlying schizophrenia. Conversely, the middle-aged woman who exhibits mild depression after a hysterectomy rarely has a serious psychiatric problem, mainly because she is past the age when this makes an appearance. Even getting older has its good points.

One cannot deny that problems do occur. But if you ask a gynecologist how many major cases of emotional depression following hysterectomy he has had, he is likely to tell you that of several thousand operations performed, he can count the number on one hand. Perhaps he will also confirm that, of that handful, most had psychological insecurities of one sort or another long before the operation. Yet writers continue to emphasize the frequency and the severity of posthysterectomy depression.

Recently, one went so far as to say that women can lose an arm, a leg, a kidney, or a lung with greater assurance than they can submit to a hysterectomy. I agree that the uterus has more psychological significance than the gallbladder or the kidney, but after practicing gynecology for twenty years and closely observing the emotional aspects of this operation on my patients, I have never seen a single woman who would rather have her leg amputated than have a hysterectomy. Some writers have simply over-played their hand in dealing with the psychology of hys-terectomy depression, particularly for modern women. Their comments are far removed from the reality of what actually transpires in a gynecologist's office day after day.

☙ BEFORE THE HYSTERECTOMY

Even in the liberated 1970s, a book on hysterectomy can-not sweep the emotional aspects of the operation quietly under the rug. Severe psychiatric problems are rare. Others are becoming less frequent. But a lack of under-standing, sometimes sheer anatomical ignorance, and the recent scrutiny of the motives for the surgery still take their emotional toll on women. Frequently the trouble results from a combination of factors. The operation comes at a vulnerable point in most women's lives and may coincide with other emotional stresses—strained marriages, prob-lems with adolescent or grown children, children leaving home, and husbands going through their own midlife cri-ses. And each morning the mirror shows the relentless pas-sage of time. Adding a hysterectomy to these underlying worries is sometimes enough to tip the balance. The route of least resistance is to blame the surgery.

It is not a new concept to connect the uterus with female problems. Plato was convinced that the womb could become discontented and angry, and, in return, cause a variety of diseases. But Krafft-Ebing, in 1890, was the first to state that mental problems are caused more frequently by hysterectomy than by any other surgical procedure. And in 1892 even the dictionary placed its stamp of disapproval on this operation. Hack Tuke's *Dictionary of Psychological Medicine* of that year stated: "To unsex a woman is surely to maim or affect injuriously the integrity of her nervous system." For decades followers of Freud have looked upon women as "castrated males" who suffer from "penis envy." This is a ridiculous concept, and most of today's women would consider it as antiquated as the one that portrays them as witless housewives who cannot compete successfully with men in the male-dominated business world. These age-old concepts are dead, and no longer do women and physicians assume that large numbers of patients will suffer from emotional troubles following a hysterectomy.

What has happened in recent years is a realistic appraisal of what may precipitate problems and how they can be prevented. Doctors agree there is a greater chance of significant depression after a hysterectomy than following other operations. For example, some studies have shown that psychological problems can be expected to occur anywhere from two to three times more often after a hysterectomy than following the removal of the gallbladder. Psychiatrists say that the emotional importance of the uterus to the patient depends on both the conscious and the unconscious ideas that each woman has about her female organs. Every woman, in effect, has a realistic opinion of how the uterus functions, but her mind is also clouded by unrealistic assumptions derived from past experiences. It is the interaction between these realistic and unrealistic concepts that determines the intensity of her fears when a hysterectomy is suggested.

Psychiatrists also stress that there is no evidence to

support the theory that, in an era of women's liberation, women regard their femaleness with reluctance and disdain. Rather, they value their femininity, so that some women with weak sexual identities may look on a hysterectomy as a threatening event in their lives. One particular study revealed that certain of these women worried that, following the hysterectomy, they would be "raw, tender, and vulnerable inside." Numerous other studies have shown that women tend to associate the uterus with their general health, or consider it a source of strength. And every study has emphasized that susceptible women fear that the operation may change their appearance and have a negative effect on their role with the other family members.

In 1957, the prominent Boston gynecologist Somers Sturgis and others added another dimension to the psychological evaluation of patients. They reported that it was possible to predict with some certainty how women would react following the hysterectomy. Patients who had strong, positive attitudes about their own femininity and who in the past had proved their ability to withstand losses did much better postoperatively. Subsequent studies have shed additional information on this matter. As one would expect, young women or those who have not completed their families are more likely to develop emotional problems after a hysterectomy. So are women who view the menstrual period as a necessary function, even though it has been painful and annoying over the years, and women who are worried that their husbands may be unfaithful or that they will have "defective sexual equipment" after the operation. And if the patient looks on the hysterectomy as a punishment for her former sexual transgressions, she is headed for potential trouble. It was also shown repeatedly that women who have unrealistic expectations of what the surgery will accomplish do poorly after the operation.

M. G. Barker, reporting in the *British Medical Journal* on 729 cases, found that susceptible women usually got into emotional difficulties within the first two years after the operation, and cited three primary factors in determining which patients would most likely require psychiatric care: first, women who had had a hysterectomy when no demonstrable disease was present; second, patients who had previously been under psychiatric care; and third, women who were unhappily married.

Hackett and Weisman, in their assessment of the psychological aspects of hysterectomy, stress that how a woman reacts depends largely on how the patient perceives herself. For example, how does she feel about the loss of an important organ in her body and how does she react to pain and anxiety? Her response represents the sum total of her past experiences, her personality makeup, and what, if any, superstitions she has. The patient's self-assessment is also governed by a network of other individuals—how she reacts to them and how they, in turn, respond to her. The most vital interaction is between the patient and the doctor, along with her immediate family. But the doctor's nurse and secretary and the hospital personnel may also play a part in determining how she reacts.

Another researcher, I. L. Janis, has stated that there are three stages that a patient experiences: the threat, the impact, and the postimpact phases. By studying these phases, he is able to predict how women will react to their surgery. Janis found that patients who exhibited moderate anxiety prior to the operation had a smoother postoperative course than patients who had either marked anxiety or no visible anxiety prior to the surgery. Worry to a certain extent was not only a natural response to surgery, but also beneficial if not carried to the extreme. He also studied the difference between informed and uninformed patients. As one would expect, patients who had been given honest and encouraging information fared better after the operation. According to Janis, the second, or impact, phase is much like the moment of truth. The danger of the surgery is about to begin, and suddenly the patient realizes that her fate is to be decided by the surgeon and others. Then, during the last, or postimpact, phase, the patient has to adapt to what has happened. She has sustained a loss, and she must squarely face the issue and understand the extent of that loss. Some women at this point decide there are more benefits to be gained by remaining ill. It may be one of the few times in their lives when they have received tender, loving care, and some women hate to give it up. However, the great majority of women take a practical appraisal of their loss. As one patient said to me, "I had always hoped that I wouldn't need a hysterectomy, but there was no point in living with this problem. I've heard a lot of stories that your nerves go all to pot, but I've never believed it. Besides, I've heard so many women say they feel so much better after the operation." Another forty-five-year-old patient told me after her hysterectomy, "When you get to this age, another phase of your life is gone. I would just as soon have kept my uterus, but there was no sense fighting the operation if it had to be done. My friends have been pretty sensible. I admit I've been concerned a bit about sex and whether there will be the same sensations for me and my husband." But, she said, "I talked to your nurse before the operation and she was very positive. Now it's all over, I realize it was a needless worry. Things have been just fine."

All these studies have helped to substantiate scientifically what astute clinicians have known intuitively for many years. First, women are less likely to get into trouble emotionally after a hysterectomy if they are sure of their femininity and have mature, healthy relationships with their husbands and families. Secondly, there is no substitute for a sound doctor—patient relationship in which the physician comes across as a competent, warm human being who is willing to take the time to explain what is going to happen in commonsense, reassuring terms. And, finally, average women with average healthy anxieties usually come up the winners postoperatively.

As every capable surgeon knows, women with unhappy home situations, previous psychiatric illness, multiple operations, those who fear death during the surgery, and those with numerous chronic symptoms that can't be explained following the hysterectomy are rarely happy patients after the operation. Similarly, women who exhibit great anxiety or who nonchalantly submit to an operation without realistically appraising the reason for the hysterectomy and what they can honestly expect to gain from the surgery often find fault with the operation. The hysterectomy usually fails to meet their unrealistic expectations, and frequently the surgeon is charged with carelessness, inattention, and incompetence.

It is not always possible for the gynecologist to prevent the onset of emotional problems after the hysterectomy. Some women with too many factors on the wrong side of the ledger may nevertheless need a hysterectomy for a bona fide reason. The gynecologist cannot change the woman's social background and solve long-standing personality problems in one fell stroke. But being aware of potential postoperative troubles can be at least half the battle.

If, for instance, he suspects she has masochistic tendencies and hopes to excise her sexual guilt by mutilation to her reproductive organs, he can quickly arrange for preoperative psychiatric help. But for those women with less pronounced emotional problems, more than the usual care must be taken prior to the surgery. This requires more than the simple reassurance that everything is going to be fine. It demands a thorough explanation of what happens in the hospital, a realistic but optimistic appraisal of the risk of surgery, a discussion of what organs will be removed, whether hormones will be required after the hysterectomy, and a discussion of any other details that might worry them. For example, a patient might become extremely apprehensive if she is not told that a small catheter will be draining the bladder for a day or two after the operation. And nearly all of these patients need the reassurance that they will receive reasonable amounts of medication to ease the pain. This mixture of preoperative information and hope can do much to keep emotional problems to a minimum.

I mentioned earlier that most women now smile at the old-wives' tales that used to predict obesity, the development of a beard, insanity, and frigidity after the hysterectomy. Regrettably, however, these misconceptions still do circulate. Now and then a patient will complain to me that she has gained weight since her hysterectomy. She is totally convinced that the operation was responsible, and often it's hard to persuade her otherwise. Yet often such women had the surgery ten or more years before and don't recognize that the passage of time, poor eating habits, and lack of adequate exercise are the real culprits. There is absolutely no scientific evidence that correlates weight gain with the hysterectomy operation.

The occasional woman also worries that she may become less feminine and develop some male characteristics after a hysterectomy. Sometimes this fear is precipitated by the news that a total hysterectomy will be done, excising both ovaries and removing the primary source of the female hormone estrogen. Or it may arise when the doctor mentions the need for hormones after the operation. There is an inherent fear in the minds of a few women that hormones will produce facial hair and a deepening of the voice. This is a leftover from the past when some patients were given the male hormone testosterone for the treatment of various problems. If the dose was too large or the treatment too prolonged, there might have been a growth of facial hair. This can still occur today if heavy doses of testosterone with or without estrogen are prescribed. But the great majority of physicians now write a prescription for straight estrogen, which totally precludes the possibility of developing masculine characteristics. It is strictly a worry of the past.

Unfortunately, susceptible patients always hear about the one case in a thousand that requires psychiatric care after the hysterectomy. They don't know that these women had mental troubles long before the operation, and they didn't hear about the hundreds of other patients who sail through the surgery without a trace of emotional trouble, or if they do, they refuse to believe them. Gynecologists would have stopped doing this operation years ago except where it was life-saving if a significant number of their patients ended up in the psychiatrist's hands. The same thing applies to cases one hears about where women have a change of heart sexually toward their partners. Lamentably, many problems exist in the bedrooms of the nation long before a hysterectomy is required. To some women the operation therefore presents an excellent out. Yet it is impossible to change a healthy woman's posture toward sex, and women who have always enjoyed sex will have the same liking for it after the operation.

To some women the uterus is still the symbolic organ of female sexuality. It carries their children for nine months. The monthly period continues to remind them of their femininity. Although most women would gladly do without it, for others, taking it away psychologically removes part of their womanhood.

Jan H.'s case was a good example of this. She was thirty-five when she came to see me about prolonged, heavy periods. She had suffered the annoyance for many years. Her doctor knew the reason for it, and so did she. A fibroid tumor of the uterus had been diagnosed some years before. It had gradually increased in size, causing heavier bleeding, more pain, and considerable annoyance. Although Jan was a bright and reasonable person, she repeatedly procrastinated about the surgery recommended to her by physicians. Instead, she settled for a series of D and C's.

It was not immediately apparent why the hysterectomy was being discounted. Jan's excuses were real— heavy involvement in community affairs and the pressures of a large family. Nevertheless, she was finding it increasingly difficult to function normally during monthly periods. She complained of the inconvenience, was beginning to take daily iron tablets to counteract a growing anemia, but always, discreetly, she sidestepped the issue of hysterectomy.

Jan was an attractive, self-assured woman. One would hardly suspect her of harboring a fear of losing her femininity. But that was at the crux of the matter. When finally confronted with the fact that she no longer had an alternative other than hysterectomy, she broke down and wept.

She admitted that her periods were a terrible problem. "But," she cried, "I'm still a woman. I don't want to shrivel up. I've got a good marriage. I want to be a woman as long as I can." Jan, for all her bravado, had revealed deep inner conflicts that were tearing her apart. It required more than a pat on the shoulder to resolve them. Fortunately, they came to the surface before the surgery and could be resolved without lingering effects.

The first step was to convince Jan that the menstrual period is totally unrelated to sexuality. Its only purpose is to set the stage for pregnancy—no more, no less. It is a practical necessity for a certain stage of a woman's life when pregnancy is desirable. Superstitions about its being a mysterious, life-sustaining power are not valid. In Jan's case it was not necessary to remove the ovaries, and she was reassured by that. Strangely enough, however, she was much more worried about the monthly period than about the hormone-producing ovary.

Some men and male gynecologists would quickly conclude that Jan's reaction was sheer nonsense. But would men be any more logical about their manhood? Shaving every day is a terrible bore. Let's suppose researchers discovered a cream that, applied once, would forever remove the need to shave. Would any males sign up for it? I'd bet most of them would run in the other direction. They wouldn't think about the practical aspects. Instead, they would have illogical fears about their loss of masculinity. And if a surgeon suggested removing both testicles during a hernial repair, you would hear anguished cries. There is no doubt that the great majority of women reconcile these inner conflicts much better than men.

I've known many women, like Jan, who continue to back away from the operation because of illogical fears about what effects a hysterectomy will have. Others agree to the surgery but enter the hospital oppressed by needless anxiety. Most of these fears are due to misconceptions or misunderstandings, and if the doctor takes the time to thoroughly explain all aspects of the operation, these fears should be dispelled. But it's not always easy to zero in on the trouble. I recall one of my patients who kept sidetracking a much-needed hysterectomy for a precancerous lesion for a reason that remained obscure for several months. Finally after a number of visits she confided that her mother had died during a hysterectomy when she was a young child. This woman had a very conscious fear that her life would end the same way if she consented to the operation. It took considerable persuasion to satisfy her that a good deal of water had gone under the bridge in the last thirty years. In this interval there had been an era of unprecedented surgical and other medical achievements. It was an entirely new ball game, and it was foolish to attempt to compare what had happened to her mother to her own situation. But it nevertheless required a number of psychiatric consultations to achieve this end.

There may also be an apprehension about the diagnosis. Doctors talk a language all their own. The patient has endometrial adenomatous hyperplasia, a submucous fibroid, or cervical dysplasia. These are all benign conditions, but mention any one of them to a patient and it takes a staunch personality to be able to accept the diagnosis without some dread. It takes more than a shrug of the surgeon's shoulders to convince some patients that the condition can be cured by a hysterectomy. And some surgeons put their foot in it the moment they start talking. One may say, "You have a fibroid tumor. It's a benign growth, so don't worry about it." But the patient does fret about it. Understandably, most lay people don't like the terms "tumor" or "growth." And it does little to relieve the fear if an unthinking surgeon says as an afterthought that tumors are not always cancers. Or that he has seen only one or two fibroids over the years that have been malignant. Patients, like most doctors who become ill, usually expect the worst to happen. So don't get trapped by big names. Ask the gynecologist or your family doctor to explain the problem in simple terms.

Prior to a hysterectomy a variety of other worries may pass through a woman's mind. They are not necessarily acute concerns, but they can make her approach the operation with more than the usual amount of preoperative apprehension. Rosemarie M. was one woman who seemed to be accepting the surgery in a matter-of-fact way. She was an attractive forty-nine-year-old woman with five grown children. Her husband was a successful land developer, and in recent years they had done a great deal of traveling. Rosemarie had none of the common worries that plague so many women. She had been reassured that the hysterectomy was required only because of a uterine prolapse. She was well aware it was only a structural problem and bore no relationship to cancer or any other disease. I had no reason to suspect that an assortment of doubts were buzzing through her head.

The night before surgery I was making rounds and dropped by to see her. I thought it would be a quick, friendly visit. But a single glance showed that the usual exterior calm had left Rosemarie's face. For the first time she seemed agitated and uneasy about the following morning's surgery. She said that her husband and a close relative had just left. I wondered whether they had brought up anything to worry her. It was obvious that I had to prolong my visit to find out.

Rosemarie talked about everything other than the upcoming surgery and seemed to be skirting around the issue. Finally I told her that I felt something was causing her concern and I wanted to know what it was. At last she admitted that although she was not fearful of having the operation because her condition had been a chronic annoyance for her, she was bothered by a lot of questions she had never been able to ask me. She thought I would think her silly.

For the next hour Rosemarie finally told me what was precipitating her concern. She had a number of physical fears about what would happen to her body following the surgery. They seemed to be off-beat concerns, and she was embarrassed to bring them up. I knew that Rosemarie had always been very introspective about her body, and for this reason I had gone into more than the usual detail as to what the operation involved and how it would correct the problem. I thought this had satisfied her inborn curiosity. But now she was throwing other questions at me: "What will fill up the space in my body once the uterus is removed? Will I have an empty space there for the rest of my life? Where will the eggs go if an ovary is left in? Won't they be trapped inside my body? Won't this give me a funny feeling every month?" And so on.

During that hour it was possible to erase all these concerns from Rosemarie's mind. And I urged her never to keep such thoughts to herself again. Her case proves it is not always the common dreads that cause trouble before a hysterectomy.

✵ AFTER THE HYSTERECTOMY

A good gynecologist develops a sixth sense about psychological problems over the years and may feel something is wrong from the patient's expression or by the way she responds to certain questions. At other times how she has reacted to previous illnesses may help to put the doctor on his guard. But sometimes none of the alarm systems goes off and the hysterectomy is performed without his spotting underlying emotional trouble.

When this happens the difficulty may become apparent soon after the operation. But I've also known it to cause chronic tension for years. Flo G., one of my patients, had been very conscientious for many years, always returning at the proper time for the Pap smear. Three years before, it had shown early abnormal changes and she was admitted to the hospital for further tests. Then a D and C was done, and a large number of tissue samples were taken from the cervix. The biopsy confirmed the presence of changes that could lead to a cancer if nothing further were done. I advised a hysterectomy, and she readily went along with this decision. But I stressed that the surgery was being performed to prevent a malignancy, not to treat an existing cancer. I thought at the time that Flo fully understood what I had told her. But while I was writing this book it became evident this was far from true.

A hysterectomy was done, and a few months later Flo moved to another city. I didn't see her again for three years. She had found a new family doctor and had gone to him for a yearly checkup. He had questioned her as to the reason for the hysterectomy, but Flo couldn't recall all the details. It was for this reason that the general practitioner suggested that she return to my office for a pelvic examination. More important, he suggested that Flo ask me to forward him a letter about the operation.

Flo's examination was entirely normal. I told her this while I was still in the examining room, and I mentioned that I would write to the doctor. Then I did something I normally don't do. I asked if she would like to come into my office while I dictated the letter. I stressed in the letter that the final report after the hysterectomy merely showed abnormal cellular changes in the cervix, and there was absolutely no evidence of cancer. Consequently there was no need for any special follow-up in her case, and there was no particular need for an annual Pap smear. I have rarely seen a patient's face light up as much as Flo's did when I put down the dictating equipment. "It's impossible to tell you how relieved I am," she said. "All this time I thought you were not telling me the entire truth. I really thought you were trying to be kind to me. For three years I've been worrying about cancer."

Talking it out can certainly solve most emotional problems. But there are times when all the verbal communication in the world will not ease a troubled mind. It takes something more concrete to drive the right message home. In this instance Flo realized that I couldn't put incorrect information in the letter to her doctor. To convince some patients, a doctor may have to show them something in black and white.

In my early years in practice I never showed the patient the final pathology report. No one in medical school had ever told me this was a sound idea. I suppose I thought, in a rather naive way, that my patients would believe what I told them. I'm sure that most of them did. But I'm also convinced that a certain number left the office with an element of doubt in their minds. Just how many Flo's there were I'll never know.

Today I follow an entirely different routine when I've got good news to impart to the patient. During the postoperative checkup, I show her the pathology report. She may not understand the technical terms used by the pathologist, but that doesn't make any difference. I simply point out the word "benign," or phrases like "there was no evidence of malignant disease." Everyone understands this language, and it can save a tremendous amount of long-term worry.

If you leave the hospital and are still doubtful, make another appointment to see your doctor. This time don't beat around the bush. Be direct. Tell him you still worry that you had a small amount of cancer and you think that if you saw the final reports, it could stop this needless worry. Would he be good enough to show them to you? No reasonable physician would refuse a polite request of this kind, so even if he acts insulted or impatient, don't be put off.

Postoperative guilt and depression can surface in many different ways. I recall one patient who was convinced her hysterectomy was related to an illegitimate pregnancy that had occurred twenty years earlier. She had decided at that time there was no way she could raise and support the child, so, reluctantly, she had put the baby up for adoption. She had eventually married and had three children, yet subconsciously the guilt of abandoning her first baby had never left her. Now, two decades later, it had resulted in a severe depression after the hysterectomy.

An unthinking husband can also add needless anxiety, before or after the operation, by telling his wife, either directly or in a more subtle manner, that the hysterectomy will close the door on their sex life. This can have a devastating effect on a woman at a time when she needs the love and reassurance of her spouse.

When some patients tell me what their husbands have said, they are often so distraught that it's easy to make the snap diagnosis that these remarks indicate there will be a lot of future marital trouble. But this is rarely true. Invariably I will discover that the marriage has been on the skids for years. There may indeed be marital troubles in the future, but they won't be caused by the hysterectomy. It is just a good excuse to bring many underlying grievances to the surface. Regrettably, both husbands and wives often use the operation as an "opt out" for sex. The hysterectomy becomes an excellent scapegoat.

Looking at the total picture, significant psychological problems after hysterectomies are today the exception rather than the rule. Most informed women follow the present-day trend of accepting the operation for what it is and are not led astray by unfounded worries or illogical expectations. That is a major step in the right direction.

HOW TO GET THE TRUTH FROM THE GYNECOLOGIST AFTER THE HYSTERECTOMY

Getting the truth from the doctor can be a frustrating experience. I've known some smart female executives who can wheel and deal in the business world but who are babes in the woods when it comes to dragging the truth out of their doctors. Along with many of their male counterparts, they haven't learned the rules of the medical game. The result is countless hours of worry about whether or not they have a serious or even fatal disease.

Women are caught in a trap that is not entirely the fault of the gynecologist. There are some women who simply don't want the truth, and over the years this feeling has rubbed off on doctors. It becomes a game of "to tell or not to tell," and often results in either complete evasion or the half-truth. Not being able to obtain the truth can be a devastating affair, but there is a sure way to get the facts if you really want them.

Most women go after the truth the wrong way, either by asking the wrong questions or by asking the right ones at the wrong time. For instance, if you have had a hysterectomy for a large ovarian cyst and want to know whether the cyst was benign or malignant, it's a waste of time to put this question to the surgeon immediately after the operation. Even if he knows the answer, there is little chance that he will tell you the whole story at this point. The reason is obvious. He does not want to jeopardize your postoperative course by giving you bad news at this time. But there is another possibility you must keep in mind. The surgeon may not know the answer himself. It usually takes a few days before the doctor gets the final report from the pathologist.

A better time to talk with the gynecologist is just prior to leaving the hospital. But often conditions aren't ideal. You cannot arrange to talk to him in private, or he may be in a hurry or be called away to another case. But even if the conditions are ideal, the gynecologist may still pussyfoot around the issue. Don't worry if that happens, because there's a much better time to drive home the point that you are the type who wants the truth.

The one sure route to the truth is to change the nature of the game. To set things in motion, make an appointment to see the doctor shortly after your discharge from the hospital. If you are a businesswoman, say you need to know the truth to look after some business affairs. You are meeting with your lawyer and accountant to make certain financial decisions, and it is imperative that everyone know the true nature of your recent illness. It is impossible for the doctor to paint a rosy picture when he is aware that your days are numbered. It would be an irresponsible way to treat a patient who really wants to know what's going on. It would also be an unethical way to handle your lawyer and other financial advisers.

Another approach would be to tell him you've decided to purchase additional life insurance and need to know if your recent operation precludes it. Or you can use the "will approach." Tell the gynecologist you have an appointment with your lawyer, either to make a will, if you don't have one, or to revise your present will, and he must be aware of the true state of your health. If you go to this trouble, you will always end up with the whole truth.

10
What Type of Hysterectomy Is Best for You?

There are two types of hysterectomy—the abdominal and the vaginal—and the time spent in the hospital is usually the same. Most doctors won't discuss with their patients the pros and cons of either type. They feel that this is the technical part of the operation and therefore the surgeon's business and not the patient's. The end result usually is that most women are simply told the operation is going to be performed one way or the other. And that's that. But occasionally gynecologists will ask if the patient has any preference, and it is for this reason that I'm going to discuss the ins and outs of both methods of operation—so you'll have enough facts on which to base your decision if the choice is presented to you.

⚫ THE ABDOMINAL HYSTERECTOMY

This is the time-honored way to do a hysterectomy. The type of incision varies with the surgeon. The great majority prefer an up-and-down incision, but others carry out a transverse one in the lower part of the abdomen. Some women want this low incision so they can continue to wear a bikini without showing any evidence of the scar.

The abdominal hysterectomy is a "must" operation for certain conditions. For example, a fibroid that fills the pelvic cavity is too large to remove by the vaginal route. It would result in uncontrollable bleeding and a high chance of injury to the vital pelvic structures. And even if the uterus is normal in size, it may still be foolhardy to attempt a vaginal hysterectomy. The patient may have suffered from repeated pelvic infections, causing numerous adhesions throughout the pelvic cavity. A uterus that is rigidly fixed by scar tissue would be extremely tedious to excise through a small vaginal opening. Most surgeons will also elect the abdominal route if they wish to remove the ovaries at the same time.

The big plus factor of this method is that the gynecologist has better exposure to do the operation. Moreover, if he gets into trouble, it is usually easier to see the problem and correct it. But the abdominal hysterectomy does have its liabilities. An abdominal incision is more painful, and now and then becomes infected. It may also, on rare occasions, result in an incisional hernia. Some surgeons would also add that it has the potential for producing a greater number of adhesions.

THE VAGINAL HYSTERECTOMY

This method has been in use for many years, but, as I mentioned earlier, no surgeon uses it all the time. As the name implies, the uterus is removed by way of the vagina. Consequently, at the completion of the operation it is only the end of the vagina that has been opened.

The main indication for a "vag hyst" is a prolapse of the uterus, bladder, and rectum. In the most extreme situation the uterus will fall completely out of the vagina when the patient is standing. It is less trouble for a surgeon to get at a prolapsed uterus than it is to get at the uterus in its normal position. Also, when the uterus descends, it usually pulls the bladder and rectum down with it. Since the only way to repair these organs is by a vaginal operation, surgeons often find it easier to carry out the entire operation by this method. The "vag hyst" has therefore become a popular method for repairing vaginal prolapse.

In the United States, some teaching hospitals are more "vag hyst" oriented than others. Consequently, whether a gynecologist does a high percentage of his hysterectomies by this method is largely dependent on his upbringing. Those who were weaned on the operation tend to stretch the indications for removing the uterus this way. Some become extremely proficient with this operation and will go to great lengths to prove that it is possible to remove even a large uterus by this route.

The main problem with doing a vaginal hysterectomy is, as I've already indicated, that the surgeon cannot see as well, particularly if there isn't much prolapse. To some extent the contrast between an abdominal hysterectomy and a vaginal hysterectomy is comparable to flying by day or by night. Common sense dictates that more accidents occur at night. But since the reporting of surgical complications is far from being an exact science, it's impossible to know for sure how many more, if any, complications there are as a result of vaginal hysterectomies. A surgeon can only form impressions from his own experience along with what he hears in the surgeons' locker room. Observation at different teaching hospitals also tells some of the story. For instance, I have on several occasions watched surgeons who are recognized as being the master technicians of this operation. I've seen them get into rather tricky situations under the most ideal conditions. The obvious thought always enters my mind: "What would happen if a less experienced or less skilled gynecologist faced the same problem?" There would certainly be more perspiration on the surgeon's brow. There might also be an unreported complication.

The vaginal hysterectomy is much more of a team effort than the abdominal one. The assistant has to be more attentive and aware of the various stages of the operation. He or she must also be gentle. Pulling too hard and tearing an important vessel can initiate a tremendous amount of trouble. This is where the teaching hospital has the edge. A better team effort is possible because large numbers of surgical residents are available to help at the surgery. In a small town a gynecologist usually has a variety of doctors assisting at the operation. Some can be rough and inattentive. It is therefore reasonable to speculate that complications arise that are never reported.

When I talk to other doctors about the vaginal hysterectomy, one interesting point always crops up. A great number have told me that they start out in practice doing more, and then taper off. I also recall a colleague's telling me about a certain teaching-hospital surgeon who was a strong advocate of the vaginal hysterectomy for many years—until he severed a ureter and found himself embroiled in a court case. He suddenly became less vociferous about the many virtues of the "vag hyst."

I think part of the popularity of the vaginal hysterectomy results from the inferiority some gynecologists feel toward general surgeons, who in many hospitals perform a large percentage of the abdominal hysterectomies. Fewer of these surgeons have learned the vaginal technique. It therefore gives the fragile psyche of some gynecologists a snug feeling to have their own operation. The vaginal hysterectomy continues to ring a few questionable bells in my own mind, although there is no doubt that it is an extremely useful adjunct to pelvic surgery in certain cases.

VAGINAL REPAIR AND ABDOMINAL HYSTERECTOMY

A good many women have a combination vaginal and abdominal operation. Usually such a patient has a moderate falling-down of the bladder and rectum. In addition there is a reason for removing the uterus. It, too, may be falling down, but the surgeon prefers the combination approach to the vaginal hysterectomy. Or it may be that other conditions are present that make the abdominal route the more desirable one. The surgeon first repairs the vaginal area and then makes an abdominal incision to remove the uterus.

If a vaginal hysterectomy for a total prolapse of the uterus is done, could there be a prolapse of the vagina a year later?

Patients who have a large prolapse already have major damage to the vaginal structures and the other supporting ligaments of the uterus. During the vaginal hysterectomy and repair, the gynecologist attempts to correct this trouble. It is usually successful, but in some cases the tissues are so weak that they again prolapse. Since the uterus has already been removed, the vagina is the only structure left to fall out.

Is vaginal bleeding after the hysterectomy a common complication?

No, it's a rare happening. But it is more likely to occur following a vaginal hysterectomy. Sometimes it merely requires packing of the vagina for a couple of days. Other times, further stitches are needed to stop the bleeding.

What causes postoperative bleeding of this kind?

If it occurs immediately after the operation, a suture may have slipped off one of the blood vessels. But if it happens a week or two later, it is the result of the healing process.

Can the ovaries be removed during a vaginal hysterectomy?

It is possible, but it can be technically difficult if the ovaries are adherent to other structures.

Should a vaginal hysterectomy result in painful intercourse?

The vagina has a greater chance of being shortened with a vaginal hysterectomy, which can cause pain during intercourse. In other instances pain results from the vagina's being tightened too much if the bladder and rectum have been repaired at the same time. If the vagina has been shortened, nothing can be done to correct it. But if the vaginal opening has been narrowed and is too tight, plastic surgery can increase the size.

Is estrogen needed after a vaginal hysterectomy?

The same reasoning applies to either a vaginal or an abdominal hysterectomy. If the ovaries have been removed, estrogen is normally prescribed by most doctors.

SHOULD THE OVARIES BE REMOVED?

Why is it that women who are scheduled for a hysterectomy rarely ask what is going to happen to their ovaries? In some instances the question is of no importance. In the woman over fifty, they will most likely be removed, and they definitely will be if they are cancerous or badly diseased. Conversely, the woman in her early thirties will usually leave the operating room with her ovaries if they appear to be normal. But there are situations in which the decision about the ovaries may be just as important as whether or not the hysterectomy is done. It is unwise to always leave it up to the surgeon. Such a hands-off approach can sometimes cause a great deal of trouble later on in life.

Women in their late thirties and early forties are in an "ovarian no-man's land." Even if the ovaries are normal, some surgeons still remove both of them, which causes an instant menopause. But other doctors will routinely leave them in. Why doctors move one way or the other is based on several variables, and you don't have to be a doctor to evaluate some of them. So you should at least ask the doctor what he plans to do about your ovaries. Your opinion might even have a bearing on what he decides to do in the operating room.

I recall operating some time ago with a former professor of gynecology at Harvard. He was in a rather philosophical mood and was pondering the pros and cons of what to do with the ovaries. "Sometimes whether or not I remove the ovaries depends on what has happened to me in the last few weeks," he said. "If I've watched a patient die from a cancer of the ovary, I often remove them. But if I've been free of this experience for a while, I'm more inclined to leave them in." An honest but hardly scientific approach! And nothing has happened since then to make it a more scientific decision.

Surgeons who routinely leave the ovaries in believe it is important to preserve ovarian function because the ovarian hormones are important for menopausal women. (The role of estrogen is discussed in Chapter 11.) They see no reason to remove normal ovaries in, for example, a thirty-eight-year-old woman, when they may produce adequate amounts of estrogen for the next ten years, or to subject women to the cost and inconvenience of either hormone pills or injections. If asked about the possibility of cancer developing in the remaining ovaries, their standard reply is that it's an infrequent occurrence. Furthermore, they say, if a surgeon cuts out normal ovaries to prevent cancer, why doesn't he apply this reasoning to the breasts? Cancer of the breast is more common than ovarian cancer. Therefore why not remove the breasts before they develop a malignancy?

Gynecologists who are more liberal about removing normal ovaries at the time of hysterectomy do so for several reasons. First of all, they think that comparing the ovaries with the breasts is the same as comparing apples with onions. The breasts cannot be replaced with anything else if they are removed. But if the ovaries are excised it's easy for the patient to take a hormone pill every day. They admit that most women who have their ovaries left in do not develop cancer, but they don't see any reason to take this chance when estrogen is readily available. Furthermore, during a hysterectomy the ovarian blood supply is always impaired to some extent. A small percentage of the ovaries will either become cystic or cause pelvic pain. A very small number of women will require a second operation to remove a troublesome ovary. Why take this chance? These doctors also maintain that if the ovaries of a thirty-eight-year-old woman are left in, they may not last ten years. Some may fail to produce adequate amounts of estrogen within two or three years. At this point, the woman has to start taking estrogen, so little has been gained by preserving them.

Women who have strong feelings one way or the other should tell the surgeon. I've known several patients who thought they had undergone a total hysterectomy with removal of both tubes and ovaries, until later in life when they were told they had a cancerous ovary. That's a terrible blow. And it's even worse if it happens to someone who would strongly have opposed leaving in the ovaries if she had known it was going to be done. Don't assume that the ovaries are gone because the surgeon says he will do a "total hysterectomy." This can be a misleading term. Always ask what he means by a "total" or "complete" hysterectomy. His interpretation may be the complete removal of the uterus and cervix, without any reference to the ovaries.

On the other hand, some women vigorously resist the removal of normal ovaries. They have strong psychological feelings about being more of a woman if the ovaries are left in place. And some women want to follow a middle-of-the-road approach. They do not readily accept the removal of both ovaries, nor are they happy about the future prospects if just the uterus is removed. I then often suggest leaving in the healthiest-looking ovary. The main point, however, is to communicate your feelings to the surgeon so that there are no surprises later on.

Whether to remove the ovaries or not continues to be a contentious issue, but one thing is not debatable. Regardless of what has taken place preoperatively, the findings at surgery should take precedence over everything else. The surgeon may have every intention of preserving the ovaries, but, following the incision, he finds it would not be in the best interests of the patient to do so. A good gynecologist would never allow a patient to tie his hands, so he could not have the final decision.

What would you do with normal ovaries in a thirty-eight-year-old patient?
If it were fifty years ago, I would leave them in because senile vaginitis from lack of estrogen is a terrible disability. But today, with the availability of "natural estrogen" (see Chapter 11), I usually remove the ovaries unless the patient asks me to preserve them.

Would you leave normal ovaries in if the woman were only thirty?
It's hard to know where to draw the age line. In this situation the ovaries would likely function for another fifteen years. Preserving them would save the patient the inconvenience of having to take a daily estrogen pill. The cost factor of about twenty-eight dollars a year must also be considered in some patients. The younger the age, the more one should consider their preservation. But much of my decision would be determined by a preoperative discussion with the patient. Most women in this age group would elect to keep one or both ovaries. A recent report in *Clinical Ob-*

stetrics and Gynecology advises the removal of both ovaries in women over thirty-five years of age who have a hysterectomy.

If you have to reoperate to remove a diseased ovary is it a difficult operation?

The second operation is never as easy as the first one. The ovary is usually firmly adherent to the pelvic wall near the ureter, and great care must be taken to avoid injury to this structure. It is at times a tedious task.

Do ovaries that are left in continue to produce estrogen once the menopause has started?

Yes, but in small amounts that are usually not sufficient to stop the problems of the menopause.

Is it more dangerous to remove the ovaries during a hysterectomy?

It is neither more difficult nor time-consuming.

11
Does Estrogen Cause Cancer of the Uterus?

Hysterectomy and estrogen are so intertwined that estrogen would normally deserve a thorough discussion in any book dealing with this operation. But during the writing of this book, reports appeared in the medical literature linking estrogen with the development of uterine cancer, which makes it even more important to talk about the pros and cons of estrogen. These reports became instant headlines around the world and caused the biggest backlash ever to hit the estrogen market. Countless patients called my office inquiring whether they should stop taking this hormone. Other patients who needed estrogen prior to surgery were hesitant about taking it. And some patients asked me bluntly why I had put them on estrogen in the first place.

The reverberations of these stories won't stop for a long time, particularly in the United States and Canada. Tens of millions of North American women have been on estrogen for over thirty years. They were given it prior to a hysterectomy or advised to take it indefinitely after the operation. The great majority had been placed on "natural estrogen," which enjoyed popularity because it was largely a trouble-free drug and rarely caused nausea, as did some synthetic estrogens. In good faith, women with or without hysterectomies had followed their doctors' advice that estrogen was desirable for the long-term treatment of the menopause. It's small wonder that they started to ask detailed questions about this hormone once these reports hit the headlines.

Is there any truth to the report that first appeared in the *New England Journal of Medicine?* Or is it the start of an estrogen witch-hunt? I have been vitally interested in this topic since reading these studies because I've always been a strong advocate of prolonged estrogen treatment. Like other doctors, I have no desire to lead my patients— or the readers of this book—astray. But there is little point in discussing the cancer scare unless women first understand something about estrogen.

Most women forget that the menopause is a relatively new "disease," compared to cancer, heart attacks, and other problems. For instance, women who were born in 1900 had an average life expectancy of only forty-eight years and so never experienced the menopause. Moreover, those who did live longer, or those who had had a hysterectomy, never had a decision to make about estrogen—it wasn't available until the 1940s.

Why did doctors bother about estrogen in the first place? Why did they begin to reject the common notion that the menopause was a natural process? Some of the seeds of doubt were planted by intensive tests, but the best evidence of all didn't require costly tests, merely the use of their eyes. Doctors had always known that as women age, many develop a condition called "senile vaginitis," which is a thinning of the vaginal lining that starts when the ovaries decrease their production of the female hormone estrogen. At times the lining becomes so thin that small ulcers appear and cause varying degrees of painful intercourse. This had plagued women for centuries but was looked on as a natural part of aging because doctors had no way to treat it. When estrogen became available, gynecologists opened their eyes to its various possibilities.

Estrogen has been aptly described as the hormone that makes a woman a woman. It was found to do many things. The most dramatic was the way it quickly cured the aging vagina by restoring the lining to its normal thickness. If senile vaginitis could be cured by estrogen, was it really a natural component of aging? Maybe the menopause was a disease after all, as obsolete as the Model-T Ford. Common sense also indicated that hysterectomy and menopausal patients would need estrogen for the long pull. If they stopped taking it, the senile vaginitis recurred. The menopause wasn't like an infection that could be cured by a single course of antibiotics. Rather, it was a deficiency disease—like diabetes, which requires insulin indefinitely.

Clinicians also soon realized that estrogen had beneficial general effects. It stopped the annoying hot flushes and pins-and-needles sensations and often removed the nervous irritability that for so many women is a part of the menopause. Research scientists began to come up with more interesting facts about estrogen. There was evidence that estrogen could slow down the aging process in other parts of the body. For example, as women age, their bones become thinner and more brittle and more likely to fracture in a fall. Many studies have shown that estrogen helps to counteract this problem. And there are also some researchers who suspect it may retard hardening of the arteries.

Other scientists argue that too much has been attributed to estrogen. But practicing gynecologists sometimes have an edge on test-tube scientists. They have their patients to observe. For instance, one of my patients was a seventy-five-year-old woman who had seen a number of eye doctors because of constant burning of the eyes. For several years she had been given a variety of cortisone and antibiotic ointments, but to no avail. One day I saw her for a severe case of senile vaginitis, which had added to her problems. While I was writing out a prescription for estrogen, she continually rubbed her eyes. She asked if I could give her some medicine for her eyes, but I told her I had no idea what was wrong with them. A month later she returned, saying I had cured her eye problem and how had I done it? Some eye doctors, after much inquiring, told me there were reports showing that estrogen can help the "dry-eye syndrome." Yet it is obvious that most ophthalmologists are not aware of this fact. We also know that estrogen can occasionally help elderly women who have a thin, irritated bladder lining, which causes recurrent urinary infections. Antibiotics used along with estrogen may work better than antibiotics alone.

No one has ever suggested that estrogen is Ponce de León's Fountain of Youth. It merely seems to soften the problems of aging. That is the reason an increasing number of gynecologists and other physicians have prescribed estrogen over the years. But now, with the estrogen scare in the air, many people are casting a somewhat jaundiced eye on this hormone. It is my own belief that this latest scare has all the earmarks of an estrogen witch-hunt, and I don't think it is something to worry about. In reaching this conclusion I've read a vast amount of material presented to the U.S. Food and Drug Administration, and I've discussed it with many distinguished scientists and doctors. I've also tried to do some commonsense thinking about it.

One eminent doctor testifying before the FDA in Washington, D.C., hit the problem squarely on the head. He said, "After thirty-nine years of active investigation and study, I do not know the cause of cancer of the uterus, although readers of the media now do." Another renowned scientist stated that in his opinion the statistical data linking estrogens to uterine cancer were wrong and that basic statistical principles were being ignored. In effect, he accused the doctors of rolling loaded statistical dice and coming up with the wrong answers. This seems to me to be one of the most penetrating reasons for looking at the findings with a very skeptical eye. It's a well-known fact that you can prove anything you want to by using figures. It has been done before with other problems. This time it looks like the same statistical song with a slightly different tune.

The estrogen—uterine cancer theory has actually been around for years. It first started when a special strain of mice that had been inbred for many generations developed cancer of the uterus after receiving massive doses of estrogen. Scientists shot this experiment down years ago. But once something is there in black and white, it's hard to completely erase it, even if the results of the experiments are proved to be misleading.

Another point to keep in mind is that estrogen replacement therapy (ERT) is not a worldwide phenomenon. I found on a trip to Iceland that ERT was not in use there. And English gynecologists largely treat the menopause as a natural process and prescribe far fewer estrogens than do doctors in North America. Yet women are still dying of cancer of the uterus in these countries. Moreover, American and Canadian women were succumbing to this disease long before estrogen was available. To my mind, that there must be some other reason for the development of uterine cancer is only common sense.

The proponents of the estrogen-causes-uterine-cancer theory say that cancer of the uterus is on the increase due to the increased use of estrogen. Yet a national survey covering the years between 1947 and 1970 failed to confirm this fact. But suppose one gives them the benefit of the doubt and agrees there are more cases than thirty years ago. Would it be a major point in their favor? Not really, because women are living longer, and since cancer of the uterus usually strikes women in their mid-fifties, you would normally expect to see an increase in this disease at that age.

What about the hospitals that report seeing more cases of uterine cancer? Well, for one thing, you can't compare the population of a hospital to the population at large. Hospitals and doctors get known for certain types of cases, which means that women with cancer are more likely to be referred to particular hospitals. But that doesn't prove that cancer of the uterus is on the increase. Another point to consider is whether the diagnosis is always correct. In endometrial hyperplasia there is an increased thickness to the lining of the uterus. In extreme cases it can look very similar to cancer. Just to be on the safe side, some pathologists may call it cancer when, in effect, it is still a benign problem.

One should also ask a very pertinent question: Why is

it that thirty years of estrogen treatment hasn't caused more uterine cancer than it has? If there were a direct link between the two, this would be the case. But well over 99 percent of the women who take estrogen don't get uterine cancer. This in itself is good evidence that estrogen is being damned for insufficient reason. It is also interesting that uterine cancer is rare in the early years, when estrogen is being produced in large amounts by the ovaries. Then, when the menopause begins, and the ovaries manufacture only minimal amounts of this hormone, cancer of the uterus flares up. This reversal does not make sense.

The number of women over fifty who develop cancer of the uterus is still very small—an estimated 60 in 100,000. This can hardly be looked on as an epidemic that has been caused by estrogen. It is impossible to speculate what would happen to the other 99,940 women if they were denied estrogen. Would an increased number die from coronary attacks? How many would break their hips in a fall and succumb to the surgery? No one can say, but it is likely that more than 60 in 100,000 would have problems of one kind or another. And certainly posthysterectomy patients who had had both ovaries removed would once again suffer from painful intercourse. Even today, with the ready availability of estrogen, senile vaginitis is still one of the most overlooked gynecological problems in North America. And in other countries countless thousands are needlessly putting up with it.

What causes cancer of the uterus is still not known, but until scientists come up with more answers, simplistic theories such as the one that says if estrogen is not taken, uterine cancer can be prevented, represents a kindergarten approach to the problem. They are third-inning predictions, and it's a wise scientist who knows, that early in the game, what the final score will be. Many other variables come into play as the game progresses. Sooner or later someone hits the home run that wins the game. Then everyone forgets about all the past prophecies. It's my bet that this will happen with cancer of the uterus, and then people will wonder why they previously thought estrogen could be related to it.

Estrogen will always be an integral tool of gynecology. And along with that of penicillin and cortisone, its discovery ranks as one of the major advances in medicine. Your doctor may suggest that you take this hormone for a number of different reasons—prior to a hysterectomy and repair operation to thicken and strengthen the vaginal tissues, or for the long-term treatment of the menopause, regardless of whether a hysterectomy has been performed or not. It is unfortunate that the current estrogen backlash will result in many women refusing estrogen who need it. I've even known women who have refused to take it following a hysterectomy. Even if it were the arch-villain of all time, estrogen could not produce cancer of the uterus where there was no longer a uterus. To believe otherwise is the type of illogical thinking that results from scare headlines, and it sets the stage for poor medical care. Don't be hesitant about discussing this whole subject with your doctor, and hopefully, you can reach a sensible conclusion about it. In doing so, you should remember an old adage: "It's not the things you don't know that get you into trouble, it's the things you know for sure that ain't so."

What is the best estrogen?
There are two kinds of estrogen, so-called natural estrogen and synthetic estrogen. Natural estrogen is the most widely

used, in part because it rarely causes any side effects. In contrast, the synthetic type frequently produces nausea.

Why do some doctors give hormone injections every six weeks?

Doctors give hormone injections for several reasons. Some patients don't like to swallow pills. Others keep forgetting to take them. Moreover, physicians know there are some women who believe they are getting better treatment if they receive an injection. And there are doctors who think it is a more effective way to administer the hormone.

Do you believe injections are necessary?

I can't see any medical advantage to them if the patient can remember to take a pill every day. Certainly, from an economic standpoint it makes no sense to pay for a visit to a doctor's office several times a year.

Why do some doctors prescribe estrogen along with the male hormone testosterone?

Some doctors think the combination approach has a better general effect on the body. This may be true in select cases, but I rarely use this method, as I believe the male hormone is excess baggage.

How long do you tell patients to take estrogen following a hysterectomy?

I usually advise them to take a tablet of natural estrogen every day until they're ninety-nine years of age.

Do you feel estrogen replacement therapy has no disadvantages?

Everything in life has some liability attached to it. Estrogen occasionally stimulates the lining of the uterus and causes bleeding. If this happens, a D and C must be done to rule out cancer. But usually the gynecologist finds a polyp, fibroid, or some other benign problem to explain the bleeding. In some cases, nothing is present to pinpoint the bleeding, and the estrogen is blamed. This, of course, can't happen if the patient is taking estrogen following a hysterectomy.

Why do some women take estrogen every day and others only three weeks out of four?

Even prior to the reports linking estrogen to cancer of the uterus, many doctors favored the intermittent routine. The rationale was that the continuous stimulation of the uterine lining was more likely to cause postmenopausal bleeding. A week off estrogen would give the endometrial lining a rest. In my experience it never worked that way. I've used both continuous and intermittent therapy, and there has been about the same incidence of bleeding in both series. But since the reports appeared, doctors are being advised to use the on-and-off routine. The same reasoning applies—namely, the less stimulation, the less chance of developing a cancer of the uterus. Maybe it's sound advice. But this theory is subject to question. First, under normal circumstances the ovaries produce estrogen every day. Second, if estrogen causes cancer, it seems logical it will do so even if it's given only for three weeks of every month. However, I imagine in the future most gynecologists will use the three-out-of-four routine, since the Food and Drug Administration has recommended this approach.

What is the best dosage of estrogen?

This depends on the patient. As is the case with any other drug, there is no point in taking more than you require. I find that most of the time the 0.625-milligram tablet of natural estrogen is sufficient. The occasional woman following a hysterectomy will need the 1.25-milligram dosage. And a few patients on estrogen who develop slight pain in their breasts may require only the small 0.3-milligram tablet.

12
Don't Get Trapped
by the Pap Smear

Regardless of whether or not a woman
ever needs a hysterectomy, she must know of the great
benefits of the Pap cancer smear. But she should be
equally aware of its pitfalls. Unfortunately, the smear often
causes needless worry. And it can also, at times, give a
sense of false security that could cost a woman her life.
This section will prevent you from falling into this kind of
trap. When the doctor says everything is fine at the annual
checkup, most women breathe a sigh of relief. But now
and then this reassurance is suddenly shattered afterward
by a telephone call from the doctor's office. The nurse
reports that the Pap smear was abnormal and the gynecologist must see the patient again. Invariably the patient in-
terprets the news as meaning she has cancer, and the wait
to see the doctor becomes one of the longest and most
fearful of her life. Sometimes this kind of call comes after
the gynecologist has advised a hysterectomy for a benign

problem. The patient immediately doubts the doctor's word or even his competence. Yet in most instances this is the wrong conclusion, and all the worry could be avoided by a fuller understanding of the Pap smear.

Some diseases hit you quickly. One day you're feeling top-drawer, and the next day it's a struggle to get out of bed. But cancer of the female organs isn't like the flu and other acute diseases. It's a gradual process that slowly changes from white to black. Cancer of the cervix, which the Pap smear is primarily designed to detect, may, for example, take as long as ten years to become a full-blown cancer. The high accuracy of the test is one of its strong points. Yet, ironically, it is also the very thing that often causes so much worry. The test is so sensitive that it actually picks up cancer before it begins. Looking at it another way, it picks up fear long before there should be any fear. Most women who receive a call from the doctor's nurse don't have a malignancy. They have what gynecologists refer to as a "premalignant change." The cells don't appear 100 percent normal. Some may look slightly inflamed, others look enlarged or irregular in shape. But usually there are no cells present that enable the pathologist to make a definite diagnosis of cancer. In most cases the smear merely raises the red flag alerting the doctor to the need for further tests.

To understand what the gynecologist must do, it is necessary to know how the Pap smear works. While you are reading this chapter, microscopic cells are falling off your skin. They're also dropping off the lining of the stomach and dozens of other organs. And this is what happens on the surface of the cervix. Normal cells are continually being detached, and fall into the vaginal discharge. Luckily, Dr. George N. Papanicolaou found that abnormal cells, if they are present, do the same thing. It's amazing that no one had thought about it earlier.

But there is another important point. When your doctor takes a Pap smear, he picks up some of the vaginal discharge on a wooden spatula. He also twists the spatula over the surface of the cervix. Remember the word "surface" because it's one of the strong and weak points of the smear. The smear does detect abnormalities while they are still on the surface, but it can't tell the gynecologist what's going on below the surface. If you have had a yearly Pap smear, nothing should be taking place under the surface. Since cancer of the cervix takes years to develop, annual smears detect it long before it starts to penetrate into the deeper tissues. But if you have neglected having smears or have had one only every five years, it may not be an early lesion.

If you have an abnormal smear, the doctor will suggest two things: first, a D and C to remove the inside lining of the uterus, since the Pap smear may have picked up abnormal cells from this location; second, the removal of tissue from the cervix. Microscopic examination usually reveals that the tissue changes are far from malignant. What further treatment is advised will depend on several factors. For instance, suppose the abnormal smear is found at the same time that the gynecologist suggests a hysterectomy for a fibroid uterus. It is now safe for him to proceed with the operation, knowing there is no malignancy present. A hysterectomy will also be advised if the surface changes appear to be the forerunner of a cervical cancer. But if the changes are minimal in a young woman who desires further children, the doctor may merely watch the patient closely, with frequent Pap smears.

I mentioned earlier that the Pap smear may give a

woman a false sense of security that could cost her life. It is a simple trap to fall into if you fail to realize another basic fact about the smear. Suppose you have just had your annual checkup and the smear has been reported as normal. But a few weeks later you notice slight bleeding between periods. You may fail to call the doctor's office for another appointment. Why should you when the Pap smear has just been done and it's such an accurate test? The catch is that the smear is extremely sensitive in detecting cancer of the cervix. Yet it picks up only about seven out of ten cases of cancer of the uterus. It is possible that you have had early precancerous changes occurring inside the uterus for several years. Now an early malignancy is present which has caused the bleeding, and it demands immediate attention. Remember that precancerous changes of either the cervix or the uterus normally take several years to develop into cancer. But once a definite malignancy occurs, the pace of growth quickens, and months can make a difference in the outcome. Don't make the blunder of failing to report abnormal bleeding at any time.

How often should a Pap smear be done?
Once a year is sufficient. The important point is not to become lax and let it go for several years. If the smear shows minor changes, the doctor may advise a repeat smear in three to six months.
What if one's doctor never does a Pap smear?
There is really only one answer. Get another doctor to do it.

13
Hysterectomy and Cancer

HYSTERECTOMY CAN CURE THE PRECANCEROUS LESION

Today an increasing number of women are having hysterectomies for "precancerous lesions." This is a relatively new term, and most patients don't understand its significance. To the majority of women, a cancer is a cancer, and there are no good ones. At one time this feeling was well justified, as most women were seen with fairly developed malignancies. But this negative attitude is no longer valid. More and more cancer in women is being diagnosed, even before symptoms begin, by the Pap smear and earlier D and C's. A hysterectomy will cure all of these women. In fact, these precancerous lesions actually cause women less trouble in the long run than many chronic problems such as diabetes, sinusitis, or migraine headaches. The hysterectomy has opened up a new era in preventing premature deaths from this disease.

Let's assume you are in your thirties or forties and are

told that you have what gynecologists call a "carcinoma in situ" of the cervix. What does this mean? The first thing to realize is that these early precancerous lesions always begin on the surface of the cervix. You will recall from the preceding chapter that these abnormal cellular changes may take years to develop. The second thing to realize is that the only way cancer can cause trouble is by invading the deeper tissues. Consequently, a total hysterectomy prior to this time gives not just a 99 percent chance of cure, but a 100 percent chance. The term "carcinoma in situ" means that the malignancy is still confined to the surface. In fact, it is such an early cancer that for several years some doctors argued it was not a malignancy, and they would not make a diagnosis of cancer unless the abnormal cells were actually invading normal tissue.

Or, let's assume you are in your forties or fifties and are told you have a carcinoma in situ of the uterus. This is, similarly, an early surface lesion inside the uterus. It can occasionally be diagnosed by the Pap smear, but in most instances a D and C is necessary. The important thing to remember, once again, is that a hysterectomy completely cures the problem.

Unfortunately, following a hysterectomy for these cancers, many women continue to worry that the malignancy will recur many years later. But if the final report shows it was strictly a surface growth, there is absolutely no chance this could ever happen. It's regrettable that doctors don't take the time to explain this fully and thus prevent years of needless worry.

Does a carcinoma in situ have any symptoms?
This is such an early lesion that it is often without symptoms. But watch out for spotting or bleeding between

periods or spotting after intercourse. Your best safeguard is the annual Pap smear and an early D and C if abnormal bleeding occurs.

Does the Pap smear always pick up a carcinoma in situ of the cervix?

Usually, but it's not completely accurate. However, if the smear missed it one year, it's highly unlikely it would do so the next year. Since a carcinoma in situ takes years to develop, the test should eventually detect it.

Are hysterectomies ever done for lesions that have not even reached the carcinoma in situ stage?

There are such situations. For instance, a routine Pap smear may show abnormal changes that necessitate biopsies of the cervix. This, in turn, detects changes that seem to be on the road toward a carcinoma in situ. If the woman has completed her family, there is no point in waiting to see what will happen in the years ahead. A hysterectomy may be advised to prevent a future malignancy.

Are some hysterectomies done for cervical changes that would never progress to a carcinoma in situ?

Many doctors would say so. The earlier one tries to diagnose precancerous lesions, the more likely it is that this will happen. There is no doubt that some cellular changes on the surface of the cervix are reversible and would never progress to a malignancy. In the future it may be possible to sort these out from the ones that will invariably change into cancer. At the moment this is a foggy area, and if there is much doubt, it's better for the doctor to be on the safe side and perform a hysterectomy. Cancer of the cervix is a serious disease, and the best cure for it is still prevention.

MADISON AVENUE
HAS OVERSOLD CANCER

It is easy to see how hysterectomy patients with precancerous lesions often misinterpret the meaning of this early form of cancer, when millions of women who will never have a cancer still have many misconceptions about it. Like other gynecologists, I see more patients who are worried about cancer than anything else. But the great majority don't have cancer. They merely constitute the growing number of women who have joined the "cancerphobia club." In our zeal to stamp out this disease, one can question whether we have oversold the product. No one would want to curtail the millions being spent attempting to solve the riddle, but have we poured too much money into Madison Avenue–type advertising selling recognition of the early signs of cancer? Is this getting women to the doctor earlier? Or is it merely creating a nation of hypochondriacs?

How did all the hypochondria begin? To some extent, it has always been there. Cancer is a devastating disease when it gets out of hand. Anyone who has seen a loved one die a lingering death from cancer is only too aware of the suffering of the patient. And of the mental anguish to the entire family. But not all people have been that close to cancer. Why does it strike such fear into their hearts? One reason is that cancer has become big business. It is an established fact that Madison Avenue can sell anything if given enough money. And untold millions of dollars have enabled their message to reach into nearly every household in the nation.

The theme has always been the same. Abnormal bleeding, lumps, discharge, ulcers that fail to heal, and a persistent cough are all signs of cancer. Get to the doctor before it is too late. I'm not saying this is bad advice. No gynecologist would argue against it. But, like a hot tip on the stock market, it doesn't tell the whole story. And it affects women adversely in two ways. One group of women (and men make the same mistake) overreacts to cancer. Let any of these symptoms appear and they are convinced they have cancer. Time and time again they rush to the doctor's office. Repeatedly they are told they do not have cancer. A good many of them refuse to believe it and live out their lives in constant fear. The other group underreacts. The bleeding pattern changes, a lump appears, and weeks or months go by before they finally seek help because they are unable to face what it might be.

What trap have these women fallen into? They've made the same error as a student at the Harvard Medical School did who was making rounds one day with a surgeon noted for his common sense. A patient had been admitted to the hospital complaining of right-sided pain, vomiting, and a slight temperature. The surgeon asked the student to list the problems that could cause these symptoms. The first disease he mentioned was cancer of the bowel. Before he could proceed further, the surgeon said, "If you walked out of your home and saw water on the road, what would you think had happened?" Somewhat shaken by the interruption, the student replied that he would think it had rained. "Correct," the surgeon replied. "Ninety-nine percent of the time that would be the right assumption, not that a fire engine had flooded the street. Why not use the same commonsense thinking in this case?

The most likely diagnosis is appendicitis, not a malignancy of the bowel. Think of common things first." Patients should get into the same habit.

It's rather ironic that one has to direct some of the blame at the American Cancer Society. No one would disagree that thousands of these dedicated people have done much to aid cancer research and have been of inestimable help to cancer patients. But even dedicated people can make mistakes. They can try too hard. Many years ago Pavlov conditioned his dog to increase his gastric fluids when the dinner bell rang. In like fashion, the American Cancer Society has trained too many women to jump to the wrong conclusion about the warning signs of cancer. Rectal bleeding is indeed a sign of cancer. But it is usually due to hemorrhoids. Abnormal vaginal bleeding can be the result of a malignancy. Yet it normally turns out to be a benign problem. And vaginal discharge is the result of cancer once in every few thousand cases. Moreover, there is still a tremendous amount of ignorance about cancer in spite of the American Cancer Society's massive campaign. Some people believe the disease is infectious. In one survey, one person in four thought cancer was incurable.

Fortunately, the American Cancer Society is following the political approach. They've decided it's time for a change. The "seven warning signs" have been replaced by the "seven steps to health." It's a sensible and hopeful approach, but it won't stop all the hypochondria. It will take a cure for cancer before that happens. In the meantime, you should take a balanced look at cancer. The odds are always in your favor that the symptoms are due to a noncancerous problem. Nonetheless, get to the doctor if there is a change in your normal state of health. Just remember that nearly three times as many people die of heart disease as of cancer. Accidents, strokes, and the flu are not far behind. There are many ways to end the game.

The hysterectomy-cancer combination conjures up so many questions for most women that I will use a strictly question-and-answer format for the rest of this chapter.

Are there unnecessary hysterectomies for pelvic cancer?

Generally speaking, the answer is no. This is one area where the hysterectomy is a much-needed operation. The one doubtful area is in the pelvic exenteration operation. I will go into this very radical type of surgery for cancer later on.

Is a hysterectomy a better way to treat cancer than radiation?

There is no yes-or-no answer to this question. The choice of treatment depends on the type of cancer and how long it has been present.

Do pelvic cancers appear at any particular age?

Cancer of the cervix is most common in the mid-forties. Uterine and ovarian cancers are more likely to start after the menopause.

Is twenty-seven years of age young to get a carcinoma in situ of the cervix?

In the days prior to the Pap smear, this early change would have been missed by the doctor, and in all probability it would have resulted in a full-blown cancer of the cervix by the time the woman was in her mid-thirties. This is still an early age for a woman to be faced with trouble of this kind, but these surface cancers are one of the bright spots in cancer treatment. A hysterectomy will cure 100 percent of these cases.

Is bleeding after intercourse of any importance?
Most likely it's due to a very common condition called "chronic cervicitis," a rawness at the entrance to the uterus. It's an area that's often struck during intercourse, and if so, it may bleed. Cervicitis usually results from pregnancy, but bleeding of this kind can occasionally be due to cancer. A doctor should be consulted.

My mother is eighty-five years of age and had one episode of vaginal bleeding. The D and C showed an early cancer of the uterus. The doctor says that normally he arranges for an initial course of radium and several weeks later performs a hysterectomy. But in this instance he is willing to do just a hysterectomy. What would be the best choice?
One wants to be as kind as possible to an aging parent, but one also wants her to receive adequate treatment. That is precisely the reason your doctor is giving you the choice. He wants to save your mother the worry and inconvenience of radium, for although this additional step would prolong the treatment, it would also leave no doubt in her mind that she has a malignancy. Equally important is the fact that he most likely believes it won't have much, if any, beneficial effect on the outcome. But in case there should be a recurrence after the operation, he wants you to be aware of the choice beforehand. If my eighty-five-year-old mother had an early malignancy, there would be no choice. I'd go for the hysterectomy without the radiation, particularly if she were in reasonable health and thin. But if she had a multitude of problems and was markedly obese, I'd consider radium without the surgery. Remember that at this age your mother will in all likelihood die of something else. In regard to a cure, most early uterine cancers are eradicated by a hysterectomy alone.

Is cancer of the uterus the most common pelvic malignancy?

Cancer of the cervix is the most common pelvic cancer. It is exceeded only by breast cancer as the most frequent malignancy in women. Cancer of the uterus and cancer of the ovary rank as the second and third most common pelvic malignancies.

Are there any rare pelvic malignancies?

Cancer of the Fallopian tube is extremely rare.

Do doctors have any idea what causes pelvic cancer?

Not at the moment. There are many theories, but I imagine that the passage of time will prove them wrong. Yet there are some interesting facts. For instance, cancer of the cervix is rare among members of religious groups where male circumcision is common practice. Wives of Jewish men, therefore, have fewer cases of this disease. Cancer of the cervix is also related in some way to bearing children. Nuns rarely develop it, while women with large families are more likely to develop it. There may also be a racial factor. Whites have less cancer of the cervix than blacks. Cancer of the uterus, however, is seen more frequently in women who have never had children.

Is there any chance one can inherit pelvic cancer?

It has never been proved that human cancer can be inherited. We know, however, that strains of mice can be bred that will inherit cancer after several generations. It appears that some families have a strong tendency to develop cancer. At the moment that is about as far as we can go.

Should someone who is still having periods at age fifty-four worry about cancer?

It would be foolish to worry too much about it, but it pays to be a little more cautious at this age when the periods show no sign of stopping. Past experience would indicate that such a woman stands a slightly greater chance of developing cancer than the average person. She should watch out for bleeding between periods or an increased tendency toward more bleeding. The doctor may decide to do a D and C if the periods continue much longer.

Is a hysterectomy ever advised for a woman who has a late menopause?

Not unless there are other specific reasons for the operation.

Can one tell normal vaginal discharge from that due to cancer?

One shouldn't even try to do it. It's an impossible task. Remember that 99.9 percent of the time abnormal discharge is the result of a common vaginal infection. Foul-smelling discharge is a very late sign of malignancy.

Are heavier periods just a sign of the change of life for someone in her mid-forties?

Probably it would be related to the menopause. It could also be a symptom of such benign problems as fibroids, polyps, or endometrial hyperplasia. But there is a small possibility that it is due to a malignancy. Having a D and C is the only sure way to rule out a diagnosis of cancer. In general, women should bleed less at the time of the menopause. A tendency toward increased bleeding or more frequent periods is a potential danger sign.

What about increased bleeding before the menopause?

The same rule applies. Increased bleeding at any age must be reported to the doctor.

Is pain an early symptom of cancer?

Pain is such a common symptom that even if a cancer is present, the pain may be due to something else. Most of the patients doctors see with pain don't have cancer. But if the pain is due to a malignancy, it is normally a late symptom.

Could it be a sign of cancer if one's stomach swells now and then?

It's highly unlikely if it happens only now and then. Most women with intermittent bloating have gas in the bowel. At other times the swelling occurs just prior to the period and is merely part of the menstrual swelling. Bloating from cancer is a progressive affair. Some women will notice that their clothes are getting tighter. Even in these instances it is usually the result of overeating. But the condition should be checked out by the doctor.

How often should a Pap smear be done?

Once a year is a good average. I've heard some recent authorities say that every three years is safe for certain types of patients. I don't agree. At the moment we have no good way of determining which women are less prone to develop pelvic cancer. Maybe we will before too long. But until that time, I recommend a yearly smear.

Should someone ever get more than one smear a year?

If the smear shows a slight abnormality, the doctor may advise another smear immediately or in a couple of months' time. But he may also advise other tests—a D and C and removal of tissue from the cervix. This will quickly determine whether the tissue is benign or malignant, and, if malignant, whether it is an early surface cancer or one that has started to penetrate more deeply into the tissues.

What type of cancer does the Pap smear detect?

Primarily cancer of the cervix. But it will also diagnose about 70 percent of the uterine cancers.

Does the Pap smear ever miss a malignancy?

It's a very rare happening. Luckily, the change from normal tissue to an early malignancy usually takes several years. It's most unlikely that the smear would miss these changes two years in a row. That's why it's important to arrange for a smear *every* year.

Would the Pap smear pick up an ovarian cancer?
It's possible, but not very likely.

How do you diagnose a cancer of the ovary?
Most cancers of the ovary are detected during a pelvic examination. This is another reason why the annual checkup is a sound idea. It is the only practical way to attempt to diagnose ovarian cancer in its early stages. Unfortunately, too often it's swelling of the abdomen, pain, or bleeding that prompts the patient to visit the doctor.

How do you pick up early cancer of the uterus?
The only sure way is by a D and C, which removes the endometrial lining of the inside of the uterus.

If an early surface cancer of the cervix is called a "carcinoma in situ," is this also true with uterine cancer?
Cancer of the uterus also always begins in the endometrial lining. Consequently, this is similarly referred to as a "carcinoma in situ of the endometrium." Later on, this malignancy will begin to invade the wall of the uterus. All these surface cancers are completely curable.

If a doctor feels a mass during the pelvic examination, can he tell whether it's benign or malignant before the operation?
Doctors can rarely be certain prior to the surgery. In fact, the surgeon may even have some doubt during the operation. In the final analysis it is only the microscopic examination that separates benign from malignant tumors.

Are X rays used to diagnose pelvic cancers?

Not to diagnose the cancer itself. But women who have a large pelvic mass will normally have X rays taken before the operation. The doctor wants to be certain it is a mass involving the female structures and not one primarily in the bowel, and he may also want to determine if the mass has caused an obstruction to the ureter.

Why is cancer of the cervix always treated by radiation?

Cancer of the cervix tends to spread earlier than uterine cancer. Numerous studies have shown that radiation gives the best long-term results. Patients may sometimes be advised to have a radical hysterectomy following the radiation therapy.

Is the same approach used for cancer of the uterus?

This situation is more open-ended than the other one. In the case of early uterine cancer, there is a difference of opinion about what should be done. Some surgeons routinely refer the patient for preoperative radium. This treatment is followed, several weeks later, by a hysterectomy. Other gynecologists quickly remove the uterus and forget about the radiation. They argue that with early cancer the results of both methods are about the same. But nearly all agree that with an advanced cancer of the uterus it is advisable to use radiation prior to the operation.

What about ovarian cancer?

A hysterectomy to remove the uterus and ovaries is the first step. In addition, the patient may be given a course of X-ray treatments after the operation.

What is a radical hysterectomy?

It involves removal of the uterus, tubes, and ovaries. But, in addition, more tissue around the uterus is excised, along with the regional lymph nodes. Cancer spreads along the small lymphatic channels to the various pelvic nodes. In advanced cancers you never know whether cancer has spread to these areas. The only safe approach is to remove them.

Is this a very dangerous operation?

Not in terms of dying during the surgery. But the more extensive the operation, the greater the chance of postoperative complications. For example, because the dissection of the tissues surrounding the uterus and cervix is quite involved, a number of blood vessels have to be removed. This may decrease the blood supply to the bladder and bowel, which in turn can result in a degeneration of a small portion of these structures. The end result is that in some instances fistulas form between these structures. For instance, there may be a passageway between the bowel and the vagina, or connecting the bladder with the vagina. A subsequent operation will be needed to repair these defects. Fortunately this does not occur too often.

What about radiation complications?

Regrettably, every procedure in medicine has some complications. But radiation therapy, like surgery, has made phenomenal strides in recent years. In the old days, less sophisticated equipment often caused injury to the bowel and bladder. This would result in the same kinds of fistulous tracts that I've just mentioned with the radical hysterectomy. These problems can still happen today, but they are less frequent.

Does radiation make you feel generally sick?

Radiation sickness consists principally of nausea and vomiting. By varying the dosage and spacing the treatments further apart, it can usually be reduced.

How does pelvic cancer spread?

In three ways. In the early stages, cancer cells enter the lymphatic channels and travel to the regional lymph nodes. They can also penetrate the blood vessels and metastasize to other areas. Later on, as the cancer increases in size, the cells directly penetrate the bowel, bladder, and other adjacent structures.

What is a pelvic exenteration?

For a very advanced cancer of the cervix, a pelvic exenteration is performed, which involves doing a radical hysterectomy and also removing the rectum and bladder. This leaves the patient with both bowel and urinary openings on her abdomen. Whether to go ahead with such an operation is a terribly difficult decision for anyone to have to make, for there is no way to minimize the change in lifestyle that this entails. I know of some patients who live reasonably well after the operation, but others never adequately adapt. Furthermore, there is no way of knowing whether the operation will cure the patient, and if it doesn't, then it has merely added to her overall discomfort. There is no way of being sure whether the cancer is limited only to these three areas. Even following the surgery no one can be 100 percent certain of this point, so the chance of a cure is fairly small. But for many people some hope is better than none at all. The final decision under these circumstances really depends on one's philosophy of life. If a woman believes that it should be life at any cost, then she has no choice but to proceed with the surgery. Others would prefer to live out what time is left without such radical surgery. I must admit that I tend to favor this latter approach, particularly if there is evidence of extensive malignancy throughout the pelvic cavity. I think in these instances the surgeon is primarily adding more inconvenience and pain without much hope of a cure. This may represent a rather pessimistic attitude on my part, but I think that wise surgeons, like good generals, should know when to retreat.

Can pelvic cancer be treated with drugs?
A good deal of work is being done in this field of chemotherapy, and it holds great promise for the future. At the moment, there is no one drug available that will cure cancer, but chemotherapy can often hold it in check for long periods of time.

Does the surgeon perform a hysterectomy when an ovarian cancer is present?
A hysterectomy is always done. This is because the cancer may have spread to the uterus. The other ovary will be removed for the same reason.

Are there any new developments in the diagnosis of pelvic cancer?
It's possible that there will be a blood test for ovarian cancer within the next five years. Researchers have found that ovarian malignancies produce tumor antigens that can be detected in the blood. These substances can now be found in the blood of women when they are present in large amounts. The problem is to devise a test that will pick up much smaller amounts of the antigens while the cancer is still an early one.

14
Why Some Surgeons Change Their Minds at the Operating Table

Does the surgeon always do the operation he tells you he's going to perform? For men the answer is nearly always yes. It's pretty hard to remove anything but the prostate gland if that's the reason for the operation. Similarly, women usually end up with what they expect when the surgeon is operating on a diseased gallbladder, on hemorrhoids, or on a stomach ulcer. But women sometimes get less than they bargained for in the case of a hysterectomy if they took too much for granted and relied too heavily on the surgeon's judgment.

Celia J. was a thirty-eight-year-old woman with three children. She had experienced painful periods for several years, and, more recently, intercourse had become painful and her periods a little heavier. But I could find nothing abnormal on a pelvic examination. I lost track of Celia after that because she moved away, so it wasn't until nineteen months later that I learned what had happened to her.

During the next year her symptoms increased, and she consulted another doctor. He also told her that he could find nothing on a pelvic examination to explain her trouble, and he advised a hysterectomy in view of the increasing pain and bleeding. Since Celia had no desire for additional children and had never felt completely safe with the vaginal contraceptive she had been using for the last ten years, she was not at all averse to having the operation. She entered the hospital thinking that a hysterectomy would be done, but once her doctor made the incision, he saw something that changed his mind about performing that type of surgery. Celia had endometriosis, which, you will recall, is internal bleeding that occurs during a menstrual period. This blood is literally trapped inside the pelvic cavity and causes pain with the period. In most cases endometriosis can be diagnosed prior to surgery, but in this particular patient the disease was situated in a number of locations that were not readily accessible to the examining fingers. Now that the surgeon had a specific diagnosis, he decided not to perform a hysterectomy, but instead he cut and burned away the areas of endometriosis in an effort to cure the patient's symptoms that way. The following day Celia found out that she still had her uterus, and was told that everything would be fine. But what her doctor failed to tell her was that this type of surgery doesn't always work. Nor did he tell her, of course, that, considering her age, many other surgeons would have disagreed with his choice of treatment. She went home knowing she would still worry about a possible pregnancy, but thinking that at least she would no longer suffer from pain and abnormal bleeding. For the next few months everything went along the way the doctor had predicted.

Six months later, things were going far from well, and

she returned to my office for another opinion. In order to assess what had gone on, I called the other surgeon. He told me he had decided against a hysterectomy because the endometriosis had been minimal and he thought he could cure it by the other procedure. Unfortunately this had not happened, and now her symptoms were worse than before the operation. A short time later, it was necessary for me to do a hysterectomy.

There is indeed a time to use conservative surgery when operating on the female organs, but in my opinion there is also a time when a hysterectomy is indicated to end the patient's problems. A woman who has completed her family doesn't want to have an incision for "maybe results" when another type of operation would definitely cure her. So if you fall into this category and the surgeon recommends a hysterectomy to alleviate serious problems you have, just don't nod your head in agreement. Carry it a step further and tell him that is what you expect him to do and you don't expect to wake up and find out it hasn't been done. This is not telling the surgeon what to do. Rather, it is being sure you receive from him what he has previously agreed to do.

15
What Is the Best Way to Be Sterilized?

An increasing number of women are asking to be sterilized, and there are now several techniques available, including, of course, the hysterectomy. This is a good thing because not all women should be sterilized in the same way. What is a sound technique for one may be a questionable approach for the next. Consequently, if you are contemplating a sterilization, you should know the pros and cons of each method.

TYING THE TUBES

This has always been the time-honored approach to sterilization. An incision in the abdomen of about the same size as that required for an appendectomy is made, and the tubes are tied and cut. There are minor variations to the technique. Some gynecologists, for instance, go one step further and bury one end of the tube in the wall of the uterus. Either way, it is a relatively simple operation, and although it is not foolproof, it works well over 99 percent of the time.

In most cases, with the new laparoscopy technique, this operation is now an antiquated procedure. The reasons are simple. Why make a long incision when a small laparoscopy cut will accomplish the same thing? Why stay in the hospital for several days when it's possible to leave in twenty-four hours or less? Why suffer from more postoperative pain than is necessary? Yet most sterilizations are still being done this way, primarily because surgeons and some gynecologists are reluctant to change their old ways, and also because it takes additional training to master the new laparoscopy technique.

There is one other type of incision that is favored by some gynecologists, and that is making an incision at the end of the vagina. This allows them to see the tubes, which are then tied and cut in the same way as in the abdominal operation. It is a well-recognized technique used in some hospitals and clinics, and one of its main selling points is that it leaves no visible scar. Also, patients can leave the hospital in a very short time.

Yet this vaginal technique has certain potential liabilities. Working through a small incision deep in the vagina, a surgeon simply cannot see as well, particularly if the tubes are not easily pulled into view. Generally the tubes are quite mobile and can easily be drawn toward the incision. But one cannot be sure they will be in their normal position, and what starts out to be a simple procedure can end up as a very complicated one. Although most surgeons who routinely employ this method become extremely skilled, now that the laparoscope is available this operation similarly becomes a less desirable technique.

There are circumstances when the old-fashioned abdominal incision may be preferable. For example, it may be difficult or impossible to sterilize very obese women by laparoscopy, for too much abdominal and pelvic fat makes it tedious to carry out the various steps successfully and safely. Or in women who have had multiple abdominal operations there may be so much scar tissue in the pelvis that it is safer to perform an abdominal incision.

HYSTERECTOMY

In recent years there has been a tendency for some gynecologists to swing toward the hysterectomy sterilization. There are times when this thinking makes good sense, but in my opinion it is a most questionable procedure for the great majority of women.

A hysterectomy sterilization makes sense only when there is extensive pelvic disease present or when the patient is complaining of such annoying pelvic symptoms as painful intercourse or abnormal bleeding. Moreover, if there is a good chance a hysterectomy will eventually be required, there's no point in carrying out a simple sterilization.

If disease is not present, why submit a woman to the increased risk of a hysterectomy when a lesser procedure will suffice? Surgeons who favor a hysterectomy sterilization will say that there is only a small amount of additional risk and that a certain percentage of women who have a tubal sterilization will suffer later on from abnormal bleeding that may necessitate a hysterectomy. Therefore, why not ensure that this cannot happen? It's an argument that has some facts to back it up, but I doubt that many doctors would use this thinking on a member of their own family. In a healthy woman without previous surgery, the operation that does the job with the smallest amount of risk is the soundest course to follow.

Consequently, if your doctor suggests a hysterectomy sterilization, make certain that he has sound reasons for his decision. It never hurts to ask why he considers this to be the best approach. In addition, you should realize that a doctor may recommend a vaginal hysterectomy simply because he is a Roman Catholic.

Most people would not think that religion would ever enter into such a decision, and in the majority of instances it does not. But the uterus—unlike the gallbladder, for example—is not totally immune to religion. In some instances it can gently push the patient toward a needless vaginal hysterectomy.

Today most people, including Roman Catholics, have a freer and more open attitude toward religion. Although the Catholic Church is still against contraception, millions of Roman Catholics are nevertheless using the pill. Some ease their consciences by saying it helps to control their bleeding pattern, but the majority accept the pill for what it is and have no moral hang-ups about taking it. Similarly, many Catholic doctors have no reservations about prescribing it. But how Catholic surgeons react to the pill and how they treat a surgical operation are often two different things. They may be very liberal with the pill but quite illogical with the scalpel. This is how it can happen.

A Catholic doctor can prescribe the pill and no one knows about it other than the patient and the pharmacist. But being king in his own office does not mean he has the same rights in the operating room. He may agree with you that after five children a sterilization is a wise move, yet he has no way of performing it in his Roman Catholic hospital. This may not present a problem if he happens to be associated with another hospital, but if he isn't, you may be headed for more surgery than you deserve.

It's been known for years that some Catholic gynecologists circumvent the hospital regulations by doing a vaginal hysterectomy rather than a sterilization procedure. Women who have had five children usually have some falling-down of the uterus and bladder. It may be minimal and causing no symptoms, but it does give the gynecologist the green light if he wants to use it as a reason for performing a hysterectomy. The pathologist will report the uterus as being normal, but no tissue committee can ever prove that the uterus was not falling down. They have no recourse but to accept the surgeon's word. Just how many "vag hysts" have been done to get around this religious restriction will never be known, but it must run into the tens of thousands.

In the event your surgeon suggests a vaginal hysterectomy, ask him if he is recommending it primarily as a sterilization procedure. He may reply that it's also necessary because of prolapse and this is a good way to kill two birds with one stone. If you have the symptoms of a fallen uterus and bladder, it may be the right approach. But if he states it's being proposed basically as a sterilization procedure, should you go along with it?

Some gynecologists of all faiths firmly believe that a "vag hyst" is a sound way to carry out a sterilization. Others, including the author, think this is an extremely radical approach unless there are other bona fide reasons for performing the hysterectomy. The pros and cons of the vaginal hysterectomy are discussed in detail in Chapter 10. You should read that section if this operation has been suggested to you.

❧ LAPAROSCOPY STERILIZATION

Women who are advised to have a sterilization by any other method should ask why it can't be done by laparoscopy. It may be that your doctor has valid reasons for bypassing this technique, but if he hasn't, you would be well advised to obtain a second opinion. I've known some doctors who put thumbs down on the procedure even though they had never seen one done. So don't let your doctor's personal hang-up steer you in the wrong direction. Don't listen to him if he says it's not as effective as the abdominal incision. If he takes that attitude, it's usually because he doesn't know how to do it the other way. And if someone says it's not as safe as the old method, remember to keep an open mind until you're aware of all the facts.

As I explained in Chapter 3, the laparoscope is much like the periscope on a submarine. It is inserted through a small, half-inch cut just below the navel and allows the gynecologist to have a panoramic view of the female organs and other structures. He then inserts a smaller instrument through another quarter-inch cut, which picks up the tubes and cauterizes them. When the tubes are destroyed, it is practically impossible for a pregnancy to occur. I say "practically impossible" because, apart from hysterectomy, there is no sterilization procedure that is 100 percent effective, but there is reason to suspect that, for tubal sterilization, this is the most foolproof method of all.

Laparoscopy, like any other operation, entails a small risk. This isn't generally realized in part because it's been labeled as simple "Band-Aid surgery" in the press. To be sure, only a small Band-Aid is needed to cover the cuts after the operation. But these small cuts do not tell the whole story. More correctly, it's a simple procedure for the patient and a more complicated one for the doctor. Occasional problems can arise. For example, the most tricky part of the procedure is the insertion by a small needle of carbon dioxide gas inside the abdomen to lift the abdominal wall up and away from the underlying bowel. Sometimes the surgeon has difficulty getting the needle in the proper place, particularly in obese women. With patients who have had previous operations, the bowel may be stuck underneath the incision and could be injured when the laparoscope is inserted. But these situations are very rare.

In capable hands, laparoscopy is, in my opinion, the best way for most women to be sterilized. But since it is a relatively new procedure, it's even more important that you have the right doctor. Ask your family doctor what gynecologist he would recommend for this operation. If you live in a small town, it may mean traveling to a larger center, but the end result is well worth the extra effort. But if you run into a stone wall with your own doctor, or have just moved to a large city, read the section in Chapter 5 on how to obtain "insider information." This will point you in the right direction.

I have discussed hysterectomy from many different angles in this book, and hopefully my readers should now be well aware of all the pros and cons of the operation and of the various pitfalls that trap so many women. I'm sure that I will be criticized for my approach to the subject by some doctors, who will say that it undermines the dedicated work being performed every day by hard-working physicians and further weakens the patient's trust in the medical profession. Yet this year approximately a quarter million needless hysterectomies will be done in the United States. Surely this current track record speaks for itself, and for the need of a book directed at protecting the consumer. Possibly those surgeons who are loath to inform the public would be well advised to remember the remark of Publilius Syrus in 50 B.C.: "He hurts the good who spares the bad."

Index